ANATOMY

IN BLACK

EMILY EVANS

lotus
publishing

First published in 2015 and reprinted with corrections in 2016
This deluxe slipcase second edition published in 2018 by **Lotus Publishing**,
Apple Tree Cottage, Inlands Road, Nutbourne, Chichester, PO18 8RJ

Illustrations and Text Emily Evans
Printed and Bound in China

MEDICAL DISCLAIMER: The following information is intended for general information purposes only.

British Library Cataloguing-in-Publication Data
A CIP record for this book is available from the British Library
ISBN 978 1 905367 87 0

ANATOMY

(Gr. *ana-*, 'up' + *tomia*, 'cutting')

The structure of any organised
body learned by dissection

For my parents

CONTENTS

Preface   7

I.   Head & Neck   9

II.   Back   57

III.   Upper Limb   67

IV.   Thorax   91

V.   Abdomen   111

VI.   Pelvis   137

VII.   Lower Limb   157

Glossary of Anatomical Terms   182

Acknowledgements   184

PREFACE

The reaction to publishing the first edition of this book in October 2015 was a pivotal moment in the vision I had for the evolution of anatomy and art within contemporary design. That first print run of Anatomy in Black sold out in just a few days which confirmed for me that people are just as fascinated by anatomy as I am, and if it can be framed in a beautiful and accessible way, then it can be enjoyed by everyone.

It is now over 20 years ago that I studied for my anatomy degree at the University of Sheffield, and I can genuinely say that I still find it as fascinating and awe inspiring as I did then. This enthusiasm has led me to share my passion for its complex and elegant systems, either by directly teaching medical students, or through the countless anatomical, medical and surgical texts I have had the pleasure of illustrating over the years.

After my degree I qualified as a biology teacher; it was only after seeing some of my artwork published in Sam Jacob's Atlas of *Human Anatomy* that I decided to pursue a study of medical illustration with the Medical Artists' Association of Great Britain as a way to combine my love for anatomy, teaching and art into one career.

Additionally, since 2006 I have been a senior demonstrator of anatomy at Cambridge University. Helping to nurture these vibrant young minds is a constant reminder of the importance of our understanding of anatomy and, of course, a wonderful opportunity to try to pass on my enthusiasm and appreciation of the wonder that is the human body. To me, there can be no purer or more perfect form.

The intention of this book was to frame our anatomy in a way that might appeal to medical professionals and casual observers alike, with the hope that it might inspire, pique the curiosity of, or simply draw a smile from those inclined to pick it up.

Following the release of Anatomy in Black, I've created or written subsequent books covering the niche realm of anatomy and art; Anatomy Rocks, The Secret Language of Anatomy and The Anatomical Tattoo. I also continue to bring anatomy into homes with my brand Anatomy Boutique.

I do hope you enjoy the book.

Emily Evans
BSc (Hons), PGCE, MMAA

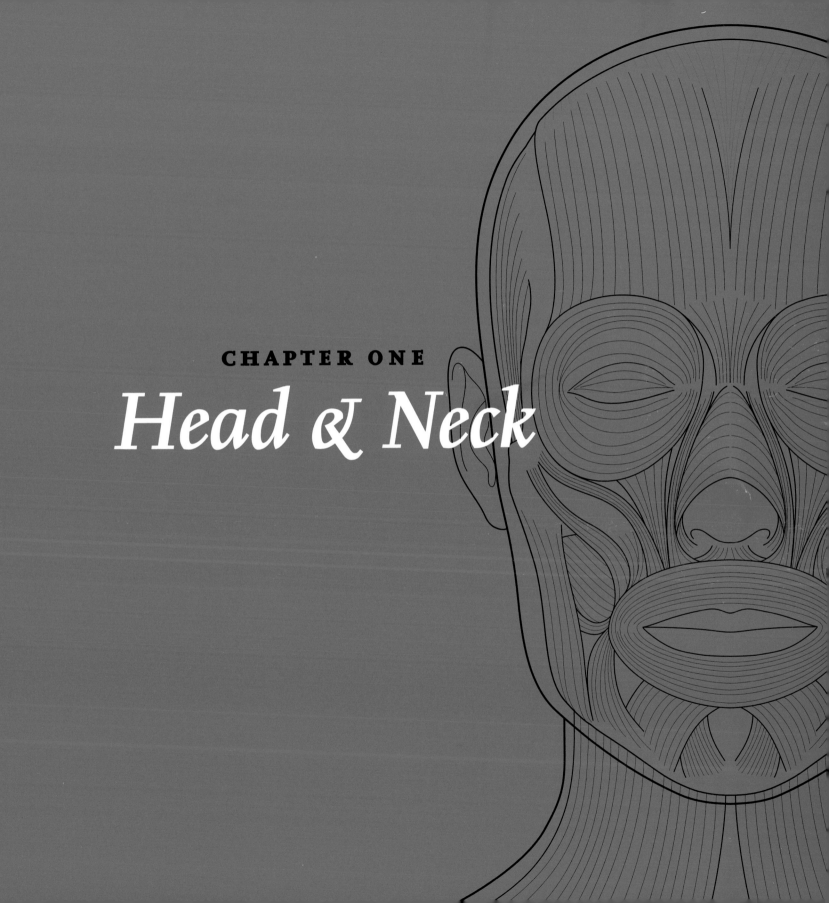

CHAPTER ONE

Head & Neck

THE SKULL

The bones of the skull provide protection for the brain and house the sensory organs of vision, taste, smell, hearing and balance. The skull consists of 22 bones in total, which can be separated into 8 cranial bones and 14 facial bones.

The cranial bones create a vault to house the brain. These consist of the frontal, occipital, sphenoid and ethmoid bones and paired parietal and temporal bones. The pterion is a potential weak area in the temporal fossa where four of the cranial bones articulate.

The facial bones provide attachment for the muscles of facial expression and those of the mouth, allowing chewing and speech. These comprise the mandible, vomer and paired zygomatic, maxilla, nasal, lacrimal, palatine and inferior nasal concha bones.

Supporting the weight of the skull are the muscles and bones of the neck. The uppermost seven vertebrae of the spine form the cervical vertebrae (C1–C7). The first cervical vertebra is called the atlas (C1) and it articulates with the skull via the occipital condyles. The second vertebra is called the axis (C2), whose projection called the 'dens' rotates upon the atlas allowing the head to rotate to the left and right.

Other than the temporomandibular joint, which is a synovial joint, all bones are joined by 'sutures', which are immovable, interlocking fibrous joints.

The cranial cavity can be separated into anterior, middle and posterior cranial fossae. The frontal lobe of the brain lies in the anterior cranial fossa where the olfactory nerves pass through the openings in the cribriform plate of the ethmoid bone. The sella turcica (meaning 'Turkish saddle') is a depression in the sphenoid bone where the pituitary gland lies. The middle cranial fossa receives the temporal lobes of the brain. This fossa has numerous foramina and canals for cranial nerves and blood vessels to exit or enter the cavity. The petrous (meaning 'rock-like') part of the temporal bone houses and protects the middle and inner ear apparatus.

The cerebellum lies in the posterior cranial fossa. This fossa contains the foramen magnum, through which the brain stem passes.

ANTERIOR VIEW OF SKULL

POSTERIOR VIEW OF SKULL

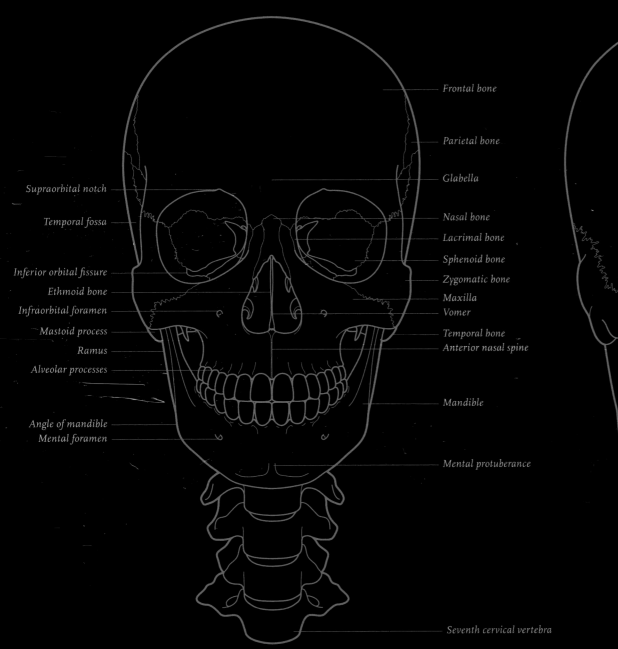

Supraorbital notch

Temporal fossa

Inferior orbital fissure
Ethmoid bone
Infraorbital foramen
Mastoid process
Ramus
Alveolar processes

Angle of mandible
Mental foramen

Frontal bone

Parietal bone

Glabella

Nasal bone
Lacrimal bone
Sphenoid bone
Zygomatic bone
Maxilla
Vomer
Temporal bone
Anterior nasal spine

Mandible

Mental protuberance

Seventh cervical vertebra

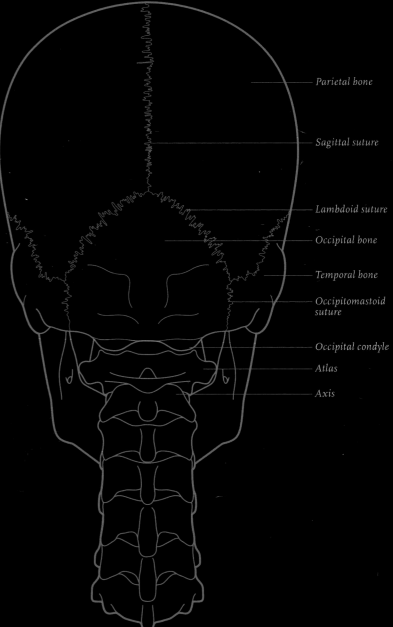

Parietal bone

Sagittal suture

Lambdoid suture

Occipital bone

Temporal bone

Occipitomastoid
suture

Occipital condyle

Atlas

Axis

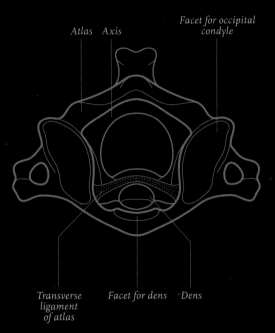

Atlas Axis Facet for occipital condyle

Transverse ligament of atlas Facet for dens Dens

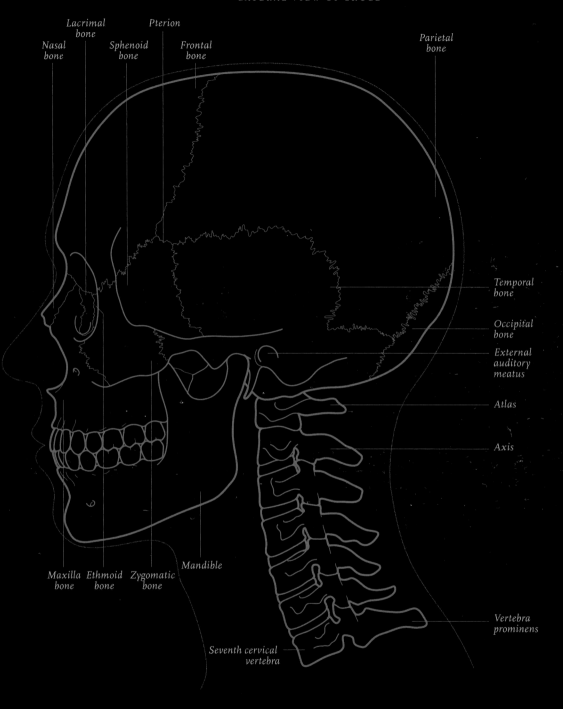

Lacrimal bone

Nasal bone Sphenoid bone Pterion Frontal bone Parietal bone

Temporal bone

Occipital bone

External auditory meatus

Atlas

Axis

Maxilla bone Ethmoid bone Zygomatic bone Mandible

Vertebra prominens

Seventh cervical vertebra

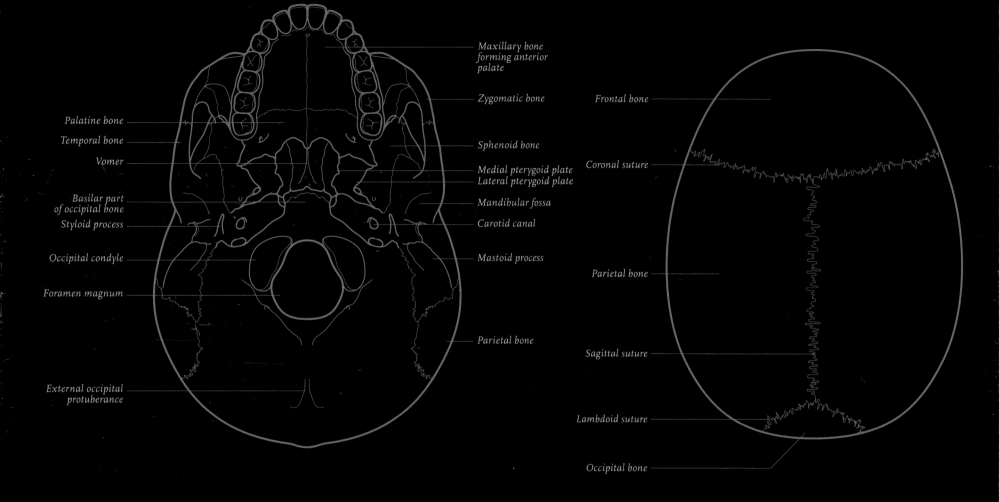

Maxillary bone
forming anterior
palate

Zygomatic bone

Palatine bone

Temporal bone

Sphenoid bone

Vomer

Medial pterygoid plate
Lateral pterygoid plate

Basilar part
of occipital bone

Mandibular fossa

Styloid process

Carotid canal

Occipital condyle

Mastoid process

Foramen magnum

Parietal bone

External occipital
protuberance

Frontal bone

Coronal suture

Parietal bone

Sagittal suture

Lambdoid suture

Occipital bone

FLOOR OF CRANIAL FOSSA

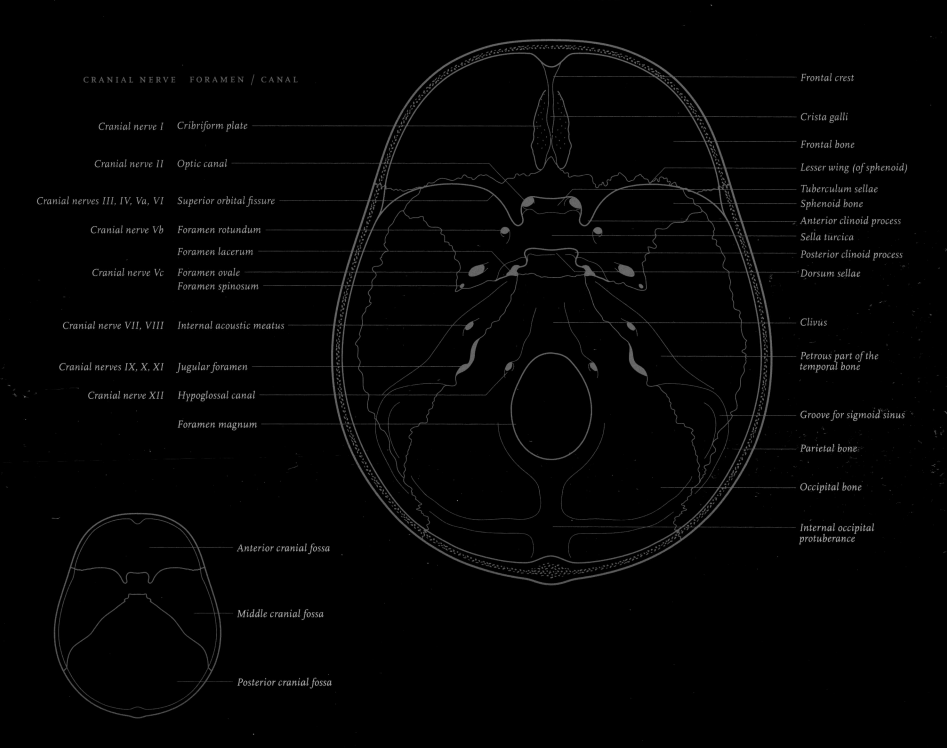

CRANIAL NERVE   FORAMEN / CANAL

Cranial nerve I   Cribriform plate

Cranial nerve II   Optic canal

Cranial nerves III, IV, Va, VI   Superior orbital fissure

Cranial nerve Vb   Foramen rotundum

Foramen lacerum

Cranial nerve Vc   Foramen ovale
Foramen spinosum

Cranial nerve VII, VIII   Internal acoustic meatus

Cranial nerves IX, X, XI   Jugular foramen

Cranial nerve XII   Hypoglossal canal

Foramen magnum

Frontal crest

Crista galli

Frontal bone

Lesser wing (of sphenoid)

Tuberculum sellae
Sphenoid bone

Anterior clinoid process
Sella turcica

Posterior clinoid process

Dorsum sellae

Clivus

Petrous part of the
temporal bone

Groove for sigmoid sinus

Parietal bone

Occipital bone

Internal occipital
protuberance

Anterior cranial fossa

Middle cranial fossa

Posterior cranial fossa

CRANIAL FOSSA DIVISIONS

THE BRAIN

The central nervous system can be divided into two main parts: the brain and the spinal cord. The brain can be further separated into the cerebrum, brainstem and cerebellum, which together form the centre of sensory awareness, emotions, thought, behaviour, movement, language and speech.

The cerebrum comprises two cerebral hemispheres, the surface of which is the cerebral cortex of grey matter, organised into a series of convolutions called gyri and sulci to increase the surface area. The areas of the cortex are named largely after the cranial bones that overlie them: frontal, parietal, temporal and occipital. The central sulcus separates the frontal lobe (which principally deals with personality, behaviour, abstract thinking, smell, speech and voluntary movement) from the parietal lobe (which is involved in touch). The occipital lobe is mostly associated with visual tasks and stimuli, and the temporal lobe with auditory processing.

Underlying the cortex is a series of neuronal tracts named white matter, the largest of which is the corpus callosum, which allows communication between the left and right hemispheres.

Defined masses of grey matter at the base of the cerebrum called basal nuclei (caudate nucleus, putamen, globus pallidus and subthalamic nucleus) have a role in helping to regulate voluntary movements.

Inferior to the cerebrum lies the brainstem. The thalamus, hypothalamus and pineal gland are all components of the diencephalon, a region at the upper end of the brainstem.

Continuing inferiorly in the brainstem is the midbrain, which is the location of the inferior and superior colliculi (governing auditory and visual reflexes respectively) and the cerebellar peduncle carrying descending axons.

The pons and medulla, together with the midbrain, contain nuclei concerned with the cranial nerves, which all emerge (with the exception of I and II, which derive from the forebrain) from the brainstem.

There are twelve pairs of cranial nerves in total. As well as a principal role with the special senses (smell, taste, sight and hearing), they also serve functions in other musculoskeletal and visceral roles.

The brain is bathed in cerebrospinal fluid (CSF), which is produced principally by the choroid plexuses within cavities called ventricles. CSF drains into the subarachnoid space and is reabsorbed from projections of arachnoid into the superior sagittal sinus.

A fibrous covering of fascia called meninges surrounds both the brain and the spinal cord. The dense outer layer of meninx, called dura mater, forms a series of venous spaces called sinuses as its outer periosteal and inner meningeal layers meet. The largest of these is the superior sagittal sinus. Folds of dura mater within the major fissures of the brain give rise to the falx cerebri, tentorium and falx cerebelli. The venous blood from the sinuses drains into the internal jugular vein.

Blood supply to the brain is via the internal carotid artery, a branch of the common carotid artery. Branches of the vertebral artery enter the cranium through the foramen magnum and anastomose with those of the internal carotid.

LATERAL VIEW OF BRAIN

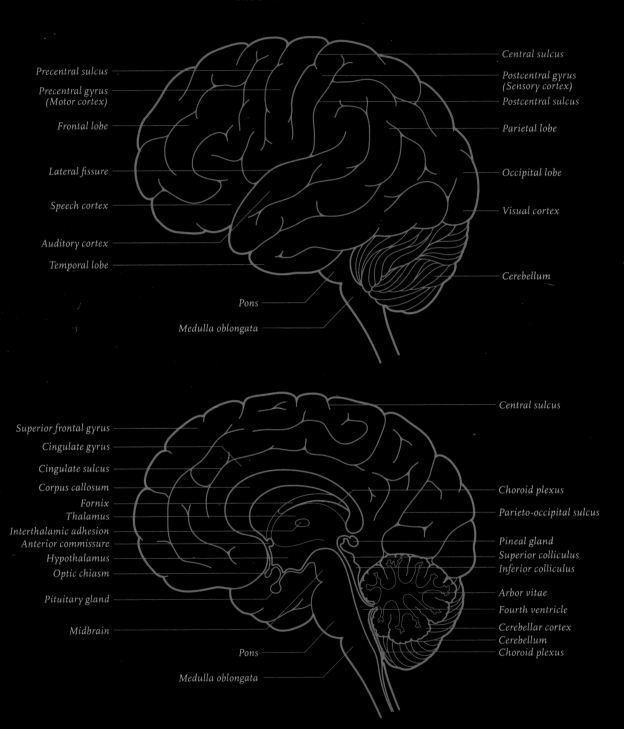

Precentral sulcus

Precentral gyrus
(Motor cortex)

Frontal lobe

Lateral fissure

Speech cortex

Auditory cortex

Temporal lobe

Pons

Medulla oblongata

Central sulcus

Postcentral gyrus
(Sensory cortex)

Postcentral sulcus

Parietal lobe

Occipital lobe

Visual cortex

Cerebellum

Superior frontal gyrus

Cingulate gyrus

Cingulate sulcus

Corpus callosum

Fornix

Thalamus

Interthalamic adhesion

Anterior commissure

Hypothalamus

Optic chiasm

Pituitary gland

Midbrain

Pons

Medulla oblongata

Central sulcus

Choroid plexus

Parieto-occipital sulcus

Pineal gland

Superior colliculus

Inferior colliculus

Arbor vitae

Fourth ventricle

Cerebellar cortex

Cerebellum

Choroid plexus

SAGITTAL VIEW OF BRAIN

18

CORONAL SECTION THROUGH FRONTAL & TEMPORAL LOBES

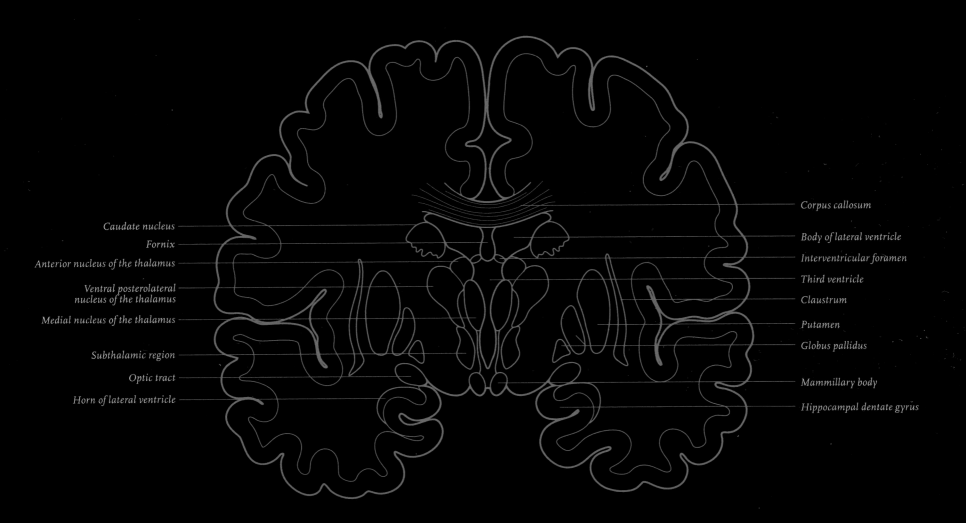

Caudate nucleus

Fornix

Anterior nucleus of the thalamus

Ventral posterolateral
nucleus of the thalamus

Medial nucleus of the thalamus

Subthalamic region

Optic tract

Horn of lateral ventricle

Corpus callosum

Body of lateral ventricle

Interventricular foramen

Third ventricle

Claustrum

Putamen

Globus pallidus

Mammillary body

Hippocampal dentate gyrus

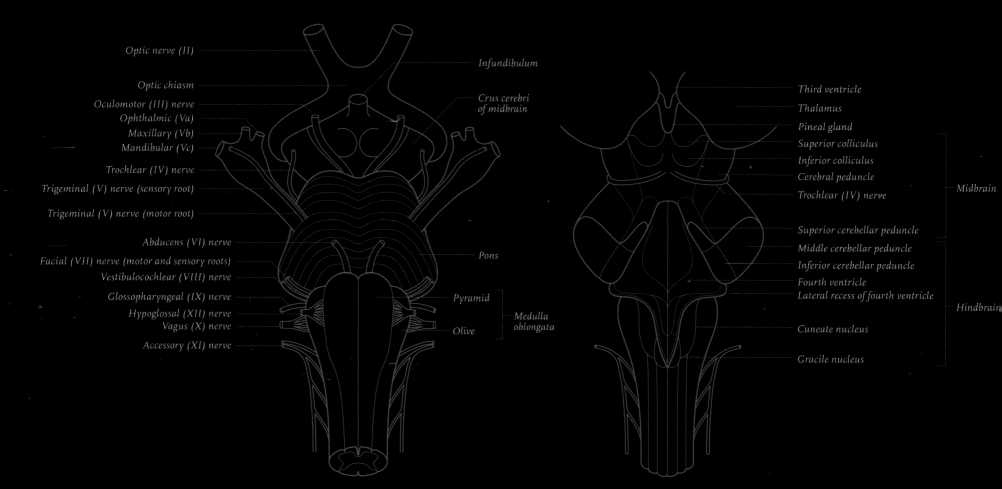

Optic nerve (II)

Optic chiasm

Oculomotor (III) nerve
Ophthalmic (Va)
Maxillary (Vb)
Mandibular (Vc)

Trochlear (IV) nerve

Trigeminal (V) nerve (sensory root)

Trigeminal (V) nerve (motor root)

Abducens (VI) nerve
Facial (VII) nerve (motor and sensory roots)
Vestibulocochlear (VIII) nerve
Glossopharyngeal (IX) nerve
Hypoglossal (XII) nerve
Vagus (X) nerve
Accessory (XI) nerve

Infundibulum

Crus cerebri
of midbrain

Pons

Pyramid

Olive

Medulla
oblongata

Third ventricle
Thalamus
Pineal gland
Superior colliculus
Inferior colliculus
Cerebral peduncle
Trochlear (IV) nerve

Midbrain

Superior cerebellar peduncle
Middle cerebellar peduncle
Inferior cerebellar peduncle
Fourth ventricle
Lateral recess of fourth ventricle

Cuneate nucleus

Gracile nucleus

Hindbrain

INFERIOR VIEW OF BRAIN WITH CRANIAL NERVES

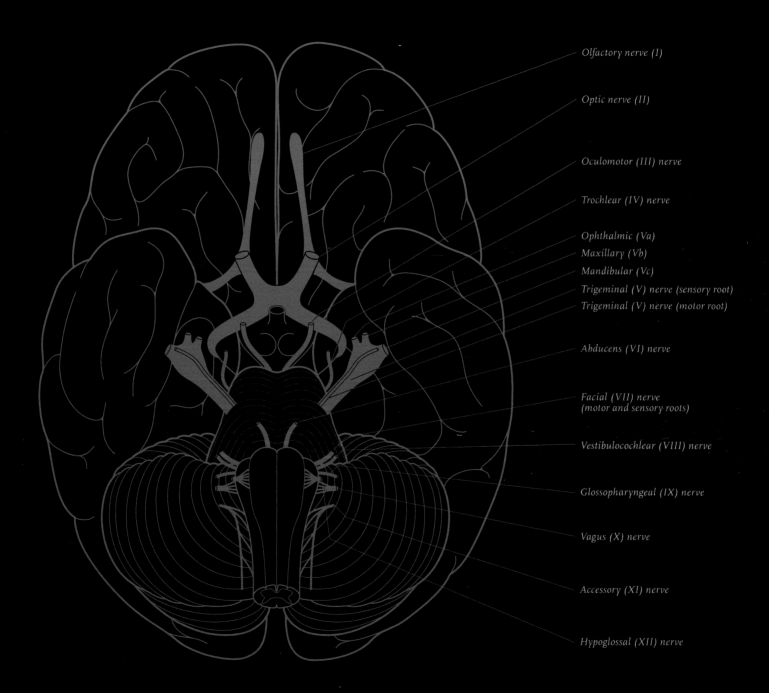

Olfactory nerve (I)

Optic nerve (II)

Oculomotor (III) nerve

Trochlear (IV) nerve

Ophthalmic (Va)
Maxillary (Vb)
Mandibular (Vc)
Trigeminal (V) nerve (sensory root)
Trigeminal (V) nerve (motor root)

Abducens (VI) nerve

Facial (VII) nerve
(motor and sensory roots)

Vestibulocochlear (VIII) nerve

Glossopharyngeal (IX) nerve

Vagus (X) nerve

Accessory (XI) nerve

Hypoglossal (XII) nerve

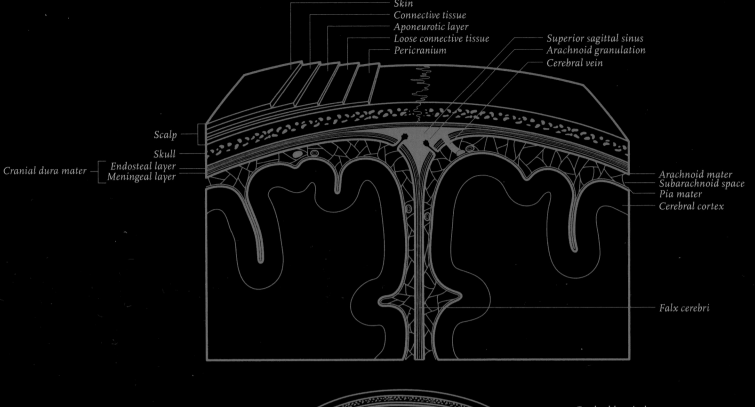

Skin
Connective tissue
Aponeurotic layer
Loose connective tissue
Pericranium

Superior sagittal sinus
Arachnoid granulation
Cerebral vein

Scalp

Skull

Cranial dura mater — Endosteal layer
Meningeal layer

Arachnoid mater
Subarachnoid space
Pia mater
Cerebral cortex

Falx cerebri

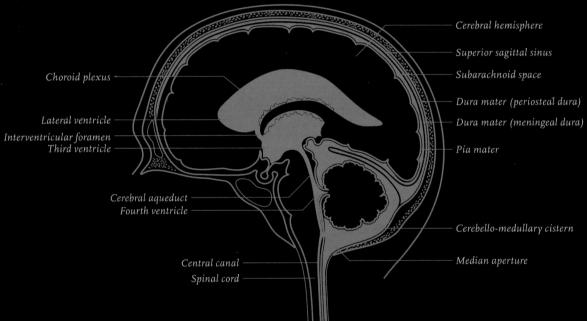

Cerebral hemisphere

Superior sagittal sinus

Choroid plexus

Subarachnoid space

Dura mater (periosteal dura)

Lateral ventricle

Dura mater (meningeal dura)

Interventricular foramen
Third ventricle

Pia mater

Cerebral aqueduct
Fourth ventricle

Cerebello-medullary cistern

Central canal
Spinal cord

Median aperture

SAGITTAL VIEW OF VENTRICLES

LATERAL VIEW OF DURAL SINUSES

CRANIAL FOSSA WITH DURAL SINUSES

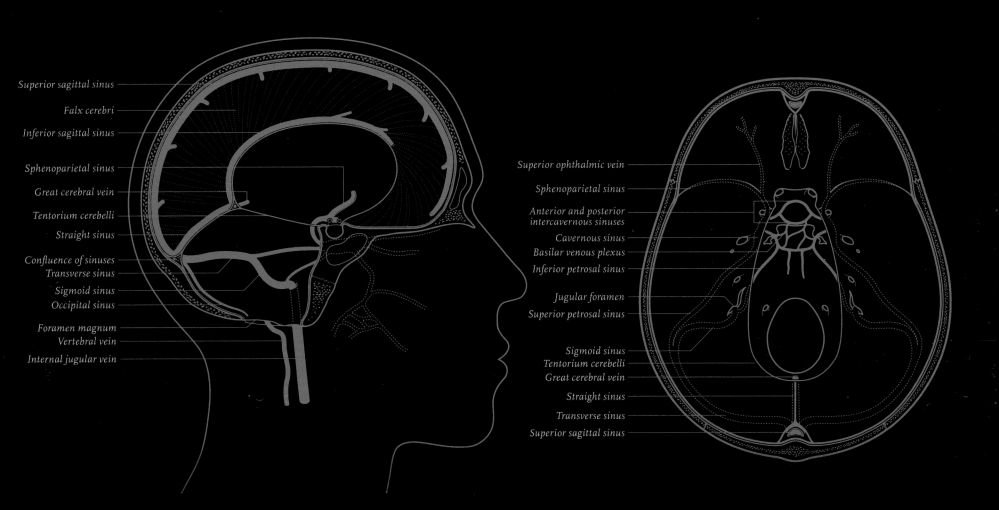

Superior sagittal sinus

Falx cerebri

Inferior sagittal sinus

Sphenoparietal sinus

Great cerebral vein

Tentorium cerebelli

Straight sinus

Confluence of sinuses
Transverse sinus

Sigmoid sinus
Occipital sinus

Foramen magnum
Vertebral vein

Internal jugular vein

Superior ophthalmic vein

Sphenoparietal sinus

Anterior and posterior
intercavernous sinuses

Cavernous sinus
Basilar venous plexus

Inferior petrosal sinus

Jugular foramen
Superior petrosal sinus

Sigmoid sinus
Tentorium cerebelli
Great cerebral vein

Straight sinus

Transverse sinus

Superior sagittal sinus

ARTERIES OF HEAD & NECK

VEINS OF HEAD & NECK

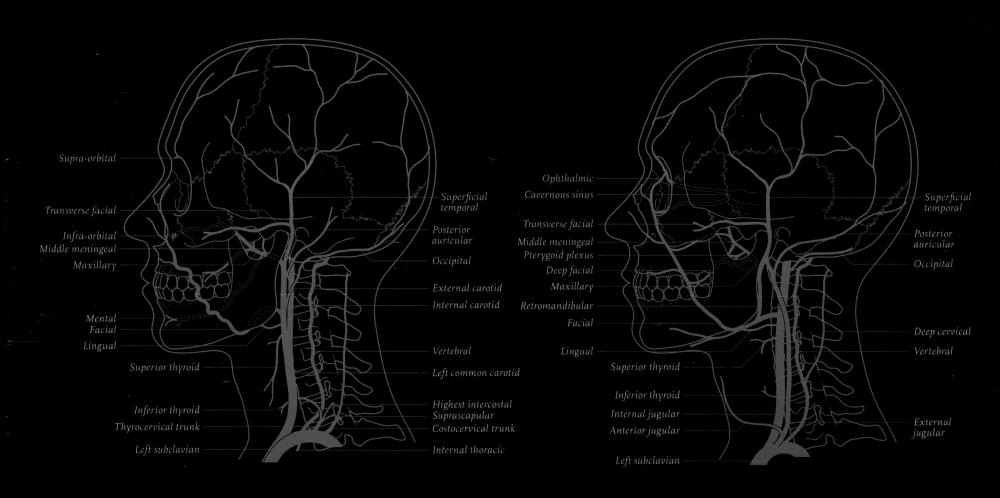

Supra-orbital

Transverse facial

Infra-orbital
Middle meningeal

Maxillary

Mental
Facial

Lingual

Superior thyroid

Inferior thyroid

Thyrocervical trunk

Left subclavian

Superficial
temporal

Posterior
auricular

Occipital

External carotid

Internal carotid

Vertebral

Left common carotid

Highest intercostal
Suprascapular
Costocervical trunk

Internal thoracic

Ophthalmic
Cavernous sinus

Transverse facial

Middle meningeal
Pterygoid plexus

Deep facial

Maxillary

Retromandibular

Facial

Lingual

Superior thyroid

Inferior thyroid

Internal jugular

Anterior jugular

Left subclavian

Superficial
temporal

Posterior
auricular

Occipital

Deep cervical

Vertebral

External
jugular

INFERIOR VIEW OF BRAIN

LATERAL VIEW OF BRAIN

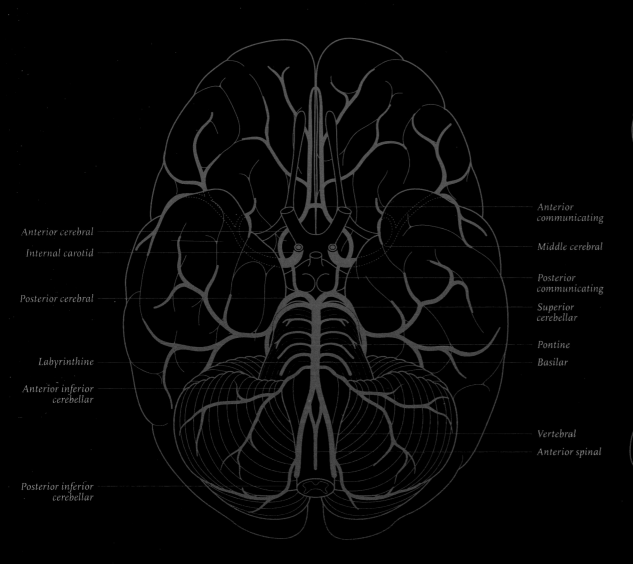

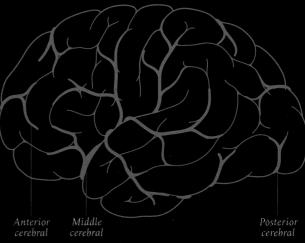

Anterior communicating

Anterior cerebral

Middle cerebral

Internal carotid

Posterior communicating

Posterior cerebral

Superior cerebellar

Pontine

Labyrinthine

Basilar

Anterior inferior cerebellar

Vertebral

Anterior spinal

Posterior inferior cerebellar

Anterior cerebral

Middle cerebral

Posterior cerebral

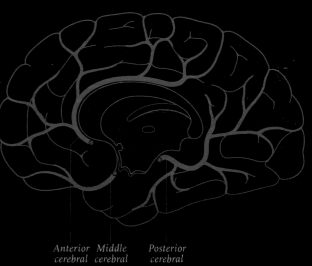

Anterior cerebral

Middle cerebral

Posterior cerebral

MEDIAL VIEW OF BRAIN

THE FACE & MOUTH

The muscles of the face are collectively known as the muscles of facial expression. Arising from the facial bones, their insertions tend to be to the overlying skin. They can be grouped into muscles acting on the scalp, eyes, nose, mouth and ears. Their actions can be deduced from their names: elevators, depressors and sphincters to close the orifices of the eyes and mouth. Nerve supply is via the facial nerve (CN VII), and sensation from the trigeminal nerve (CN V).

The remaining muscles of the face are the muscles of mastication, namely: temporalis, masseter and the medial/lateral pterygoids. These muscles act to elevate, depress, protrude, retract, and medially or laterally move the mandible. The temporomandibular joint, which allows for these actions, is a synovial joint with a central articular cartilaginous disc. Lateral pterygoid inserts into this disc pulling it forward in mouth opening whilst the mandibular head rotates in the infratemporal fossa.

Partially surrounding the masseter muscle is the parotid gland, one of three paired salivary glands secreting saliva into the mouth. The duct of the parotid gland can be palpated over masseter before it turns on the free border, to enter the mouth cavity lateral to the second molar. The submandibular and sublingual salivary glands are all supplied by the facial nerve (CN VII) and the parotid gland is supplied via the lesser petrosal nerve of the glossopharyngeal nerve.

The tongue is a muscular structure with multiple functions. The first is to move food around the mouth cavity to enable productive mastication and subsequent swallowing. It also has a role in speech, thus a complicated arrangement of movements is needed. These intricate movements are attributed to both the intrinsic muscles of the tongue (which originate and insert in the tongue), and the extrinsic muscles, which have bony origins and insert into the tongue. Motor nerve supply to the tongue is via the hypoglossal nerve (CN XII). General sensory innervation is by the lingual nerve, a branch of the trigeminal nerve (CN Vc) and the glossopharyngeal nerve (IX) for the posterior third.

The tongue is also the organ of the special sense of taste. This stimulus is sensed by the facial nerve (CN VII) for the anterior two-thirds of the tongue, and the glossopharyngeal nerve (CN IX) for the posterior third of the tongue. To facilitate the transmission of chemical taste information to the brain by the nerves, the tongue is covered in a series of papillae and taste buds.

Each adult has approximately 32 teeth. Each tooth is shaped according to its role in biting (incisors), tearing (canines) or grinding (molars) food matter. The teeth are held in deep sockets in the maxillary bones and mandible, through which their nerve supply from the trigeminal nerve comes via superior and inferior alveolar nerves. With 99% mineral content, the enamel that covers the crown of the tooth is the hardest substance in the body. Beneath this lies the dentine, which encloses the pulp cavity containing the blood vessels and nerves.

ANTERIOR VIEW OF FACIAL MUSCLES

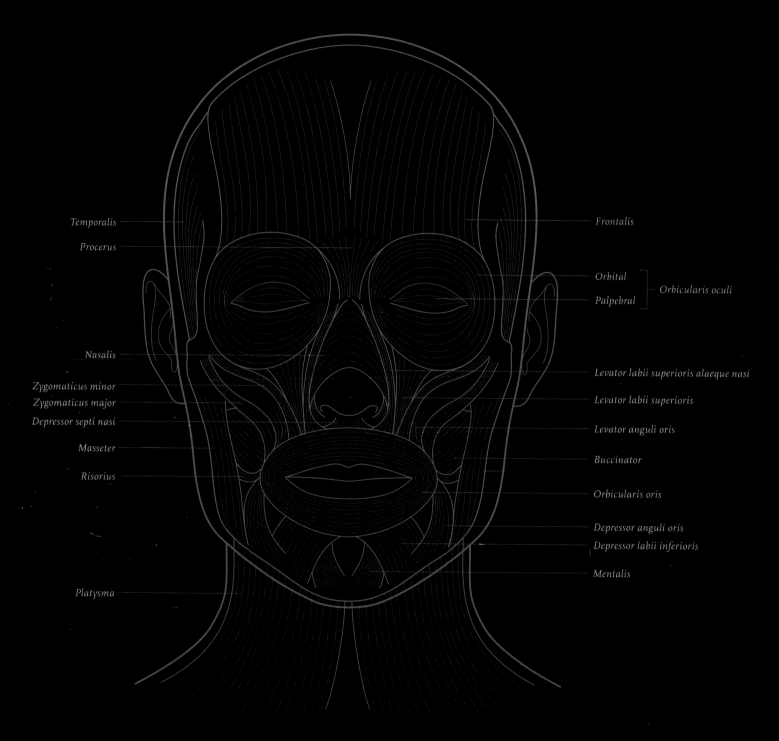

Temporalis

Procerus

Nasalis

Zygomaticus minor

Zygomaticus major

Depressor septi nasi

Masseter

Risorius

Platysma

Frontalis

Orbital

Palpebral

Orbicularis oculi

Levator labii superioris alaeque nasi

Levator labii superioris

Levator anguli oris

Buccinator

Orbicularis oris

Depressor anguli oris

Depressor labii inferioris

Mentalis

LATERAL VIEW OF FACIAL MUSCLES

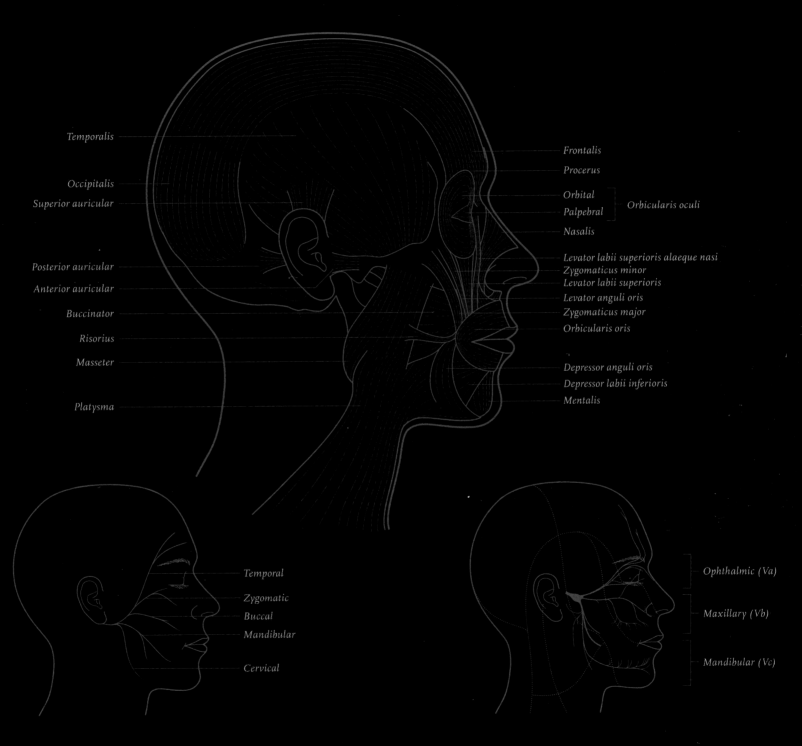

Temporalis

Occipitalis

Superior auricular

Posterior auricular

Anterior auricular

Buccinator

Risorius

Masseter

Platysma

Frontalis

Procerus

Orbital

Palpebral

Orbicularis oculi

Nasalis

Levator labii superioris alaeque nasi

Zygomaticus minor

Levator labii superioris

Levator anguli oris

Zygomaticus major

Orbicularis oris

Depressor anguli oris

Depressor labii inferioris

Mentalis

Temporal

Zygomatic

Buccal

Mandibular

Cervical

Ophthalmic (Va)

Maxillary (Vb)

Mandibular (Vc)

BRANCHES OF FACIAL NERVE (CN VII)

BRANCHES OF TRIGEMINAL NERVE (CN V)

LATERAL VIEW OF SKULL

LATERAL VIEW OF TEMPOROMANDIBULAR JOINT

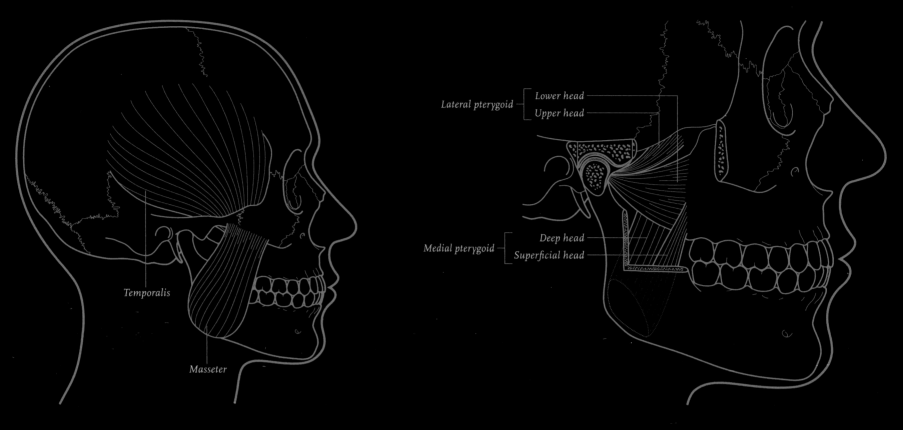

Lateral pterygoid — Lower head
                     Upper head

Temporalis

Medial pterygoid — Deep head
                    Superficial head

Masseter

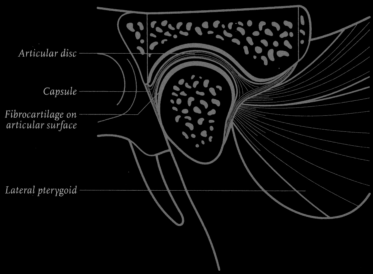

Articular disc

Capsule

Fibrocartilage on
articular surface

Lateral pterygoid

SECTION THROUGH TEMPOROMANDIBULAR JOINT

30

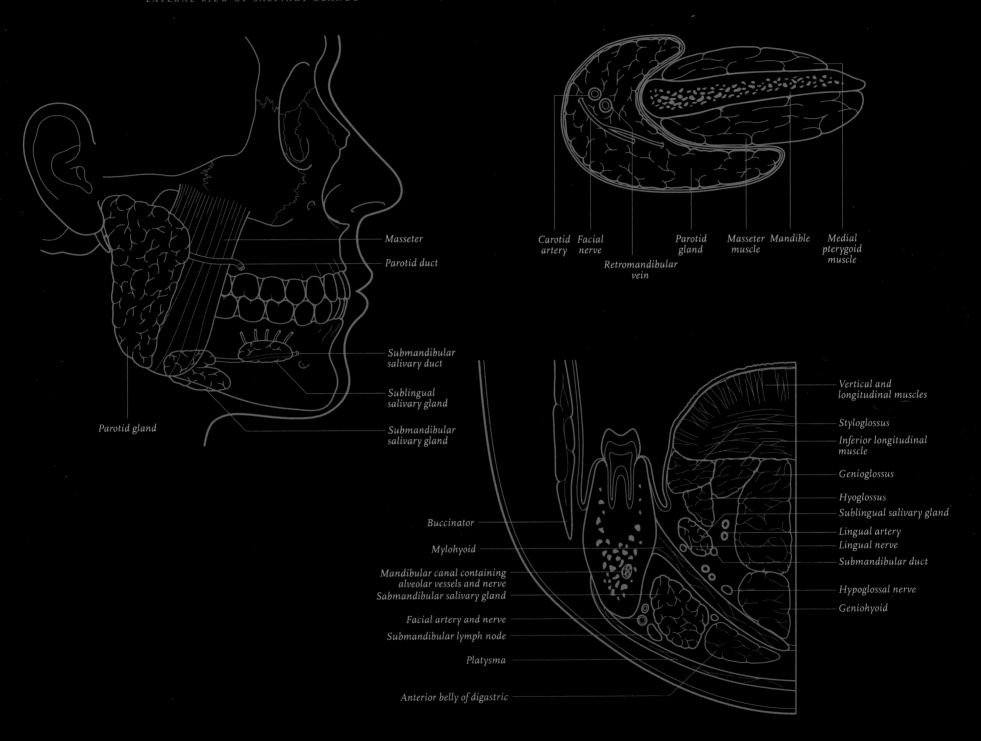

LATERAL VIEW OF SALIVARY GLANDS

TRANSVERSE SECTION THROUGH PAROTID GLAND

Masseter

Parotid duct

Submandibular
salivary duct

Sublingual
salivary gland

Submandibular
salivary gland

Parotid gland

Carotid   Facial   Parotid   Masseter Mandible Medial
artery   nerve   gland   muscle   pterygoid
                Retromandibular   muscle
                vein

Vertical and
longitudinal muscles

Styloglossus

Inferior longitudinal
muscle

Genioglossus

Hyoglossus

Sublingual salivary gland

Lingual artery

Lingual nerve

Submandibular duct

Hypoglossal nerve

Geniohyoid

Buccinator

Mylohyoid

Mandibular canal containing
alveolar vessels and nerve
Sabmandibular salivary gland

Facial artery and nerve

Submandibular lymph node

Platysma

Anterior belly of digastric

CORONAL VIEW THROUGH MOUTH

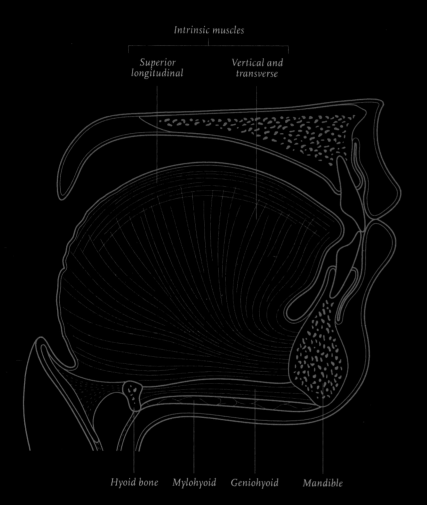

Intrinsic muscles

Superior longitudinal

Vertical and transverse

Hyoid bone   *Mylohyoid*   *Geniohyoid*   *Mandible*

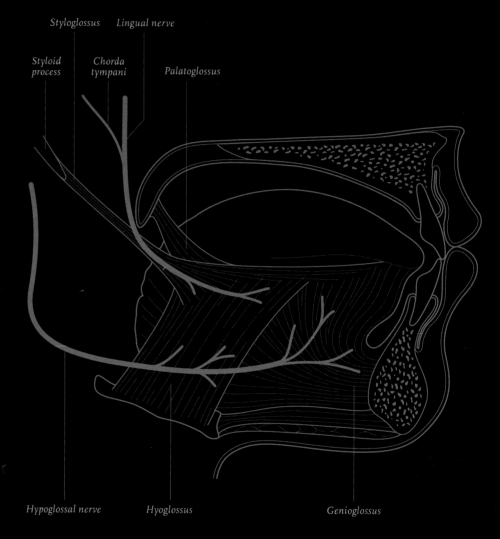

Styloglossus   *Lingual nerve*

Styloid process   *Chorda tympani*   *Palatoglossus*

Hypoglossal nerve   *Hyoglossus*   *Genioglossus*

SUPERIOR VIEW OF TONGUE

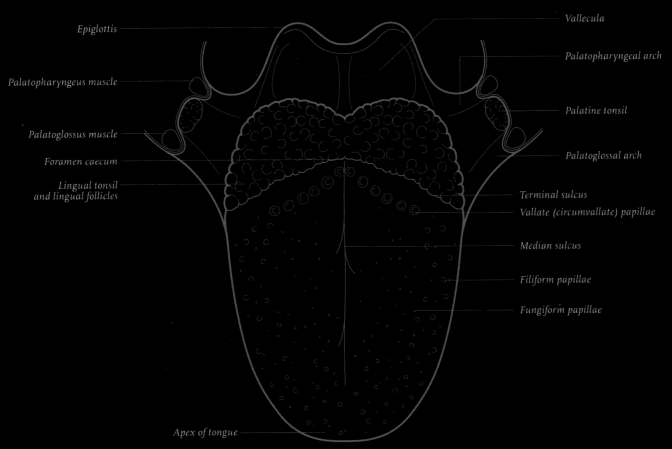

Epiglottis

Palatopharyngeus muscle

Palatoglossus muscle

Foramen caecum

Lingual tonsil
and lingual follicles

Vallecula

Palatopharyngeal arch

Palatine tonsil

Palatoglossal arch

Terminal sulcus

Vallate (circumvallate) papillae

Median sulcus

Filiform papillae

Fungiform papillae

Apex of tongue

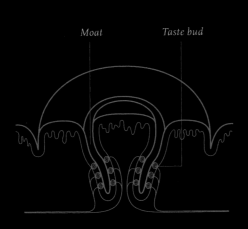

Moat

Taste bud

VALLATE PAPILLA

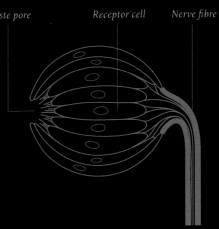

Taste pore

Receptor cell

Nerve fibre

TASTE BUD

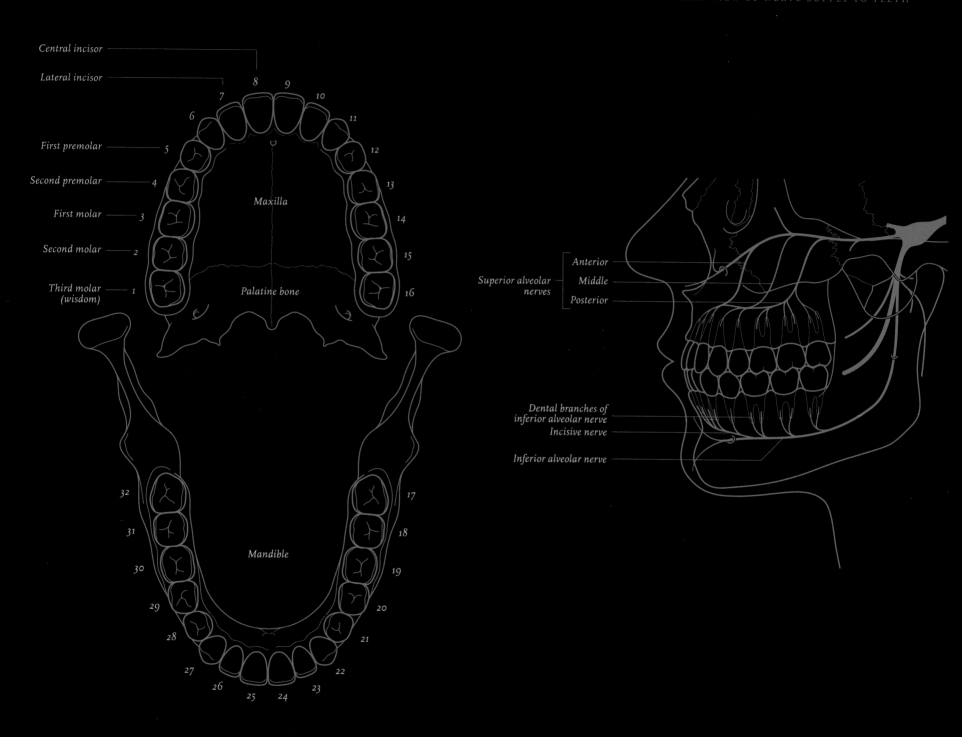

Central incisor

Lateral incisor

8 9
7 10
6 11

First premolar — 5 12

Second premolar — 4 13

First molar — 3 14

Second molar — 2 15

Third molar
(wisdom) — 1 16

Maxilla

Palatine bone

Superior alveolar
nerves

Anterior
Middle
Posterior

Dental branches of
inferior alveolar nerve

Incisive nerve

Inferior alveolar nerve

32 17
31 18
30 19
29 20
28 21
27 22
26 23
25 24

Mandible

34

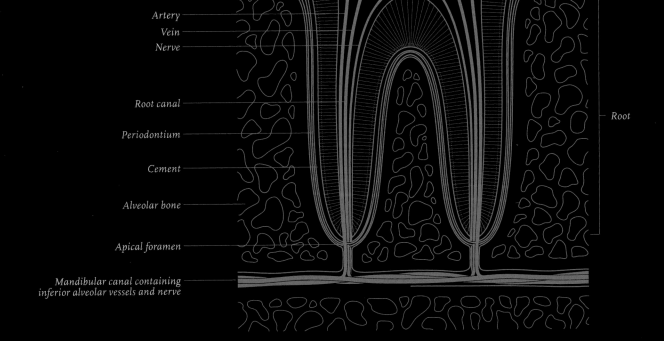

Artery

Vein

Nerve

Root canal

Periodontium

Cement

Alveolar bone

Apical foramen

Mandibular canal containing
inferior alveolar vessels and nerve

Root

THE EYE, NOSE & EAR

The eye is housed within the bony orbit of the skull. It is spherical, with a transparent window anteriorly called the cornea, which allows light to enter the eyeball. The coloured muscular iris divides the fluid-filled anterior chamber from the posterior chamber. The iris is controlled automatically, altering the size of its central aperture, the pupil, thus determining the amount of light passing through the lens. Dilation of the pupil is under sympathetic control (long ciliary nerves), whilst constriction of the aperture is under parasympathetic innervation (short ciliary nerves). The muscular ciliary body acts on the suspensory ligaments of the lens, allowing the lens to be stretched accordingly to refract the light. In conjunction with one another, the cornea, lens and aqueous/vitreous humour all act to focus the light on the retina covering the posterior wall of the eyeball.

The highly vascular retina is a membrane comprising cells that convert light stimuli to electrochemical signals that can be conducted to the central nervous system (CNS) via the optic nerve (CN II). Where the central retinal blood vessels enter or leave the retina is a zone called the optic disc that has no light receptor cells. For this reason it is also know as the 'blind spot'. Contrastingly, an area termed the macula lutea has a dense accumulation of colour-sensitive cells known as the fovea.

An arrangement of extraocular muscles facilitates the intricate tracking movement of the eye. With the exception of levator palpebrae superioris, which raises the eyelid, all the other muscles move the eyeball itself. With innervation from the oculomotor (CN III), trochlear (CN IV) and abducens (CN VI) nerves, these muscles elevate, depress, abduct, adduct and internally/externally rotate the eyeball.

The lacrimal gland, whose secretion is controlled by fibres originating from the facial nerve (CN VII), bathes the eye with tears. These are spread across the surface of the eyeball by movements of the eyelids to wash debris from the corneal surface. Tears then drain into the nasolacrimal ducts terminating in the nasal cavity.

The nasal cavity is lined with moist and ciliated (with tiny hair-like projections) respiratory epithelium. This epithelium warms and moistens incoming air on its way to the lungs for respiration. Three paired bony projections on the lateral walls of the nasal cavity, called conchae, increase the surface area for this purpose. The moist mucosa at the roof of the nasal cavity dissolves airborne chemicals to be sensed by the olfactory nerve (CN I), whose fibres perforate the cribriform plate of the ethmoid bone.

The skull also has a series of cavities called sinuses. These sinuses are lined with respiratory epithelium and are thought to lighten the skull and add resonance to the voice. They are named after the bones that house them and each one drains into the nasal cavity beneath the corresponding nasal concha. The majority of the external nose is composed of cartilage, as is the external ear.

The middle and inner ear are home to the auditory and vestibular systems encased within the temporal bone. Vibrations, known as sound waves, travel down the ear canal and vibrate the taut tympanic membrane. Attached to this are the three smallest bones in the body: the malleus, incus and stapes, connected by synovial joints. These ossicles amplify and transmit the vibrations to the inner ear through the oval window to the fluid within the cochlea. Specialised cells in the cochlea duct convert movement energy into electrical energy, to be interpreted as sound by the brain via the cochlea portion of the vestibulocochlear nerve (CN VIII).

Also residing in the inner ear is the vestibular system, a series of semicircular canals organised at 90 degrees to one another. Within these canals are semicircular ducts filled with fluid (endolymph) and terminating in ampullae. Movement of the head is detected in the movement of the gelatinous-filled ampullae, which transmit this information to the brain via the vestibular part of the vestibulocochlear nerve.

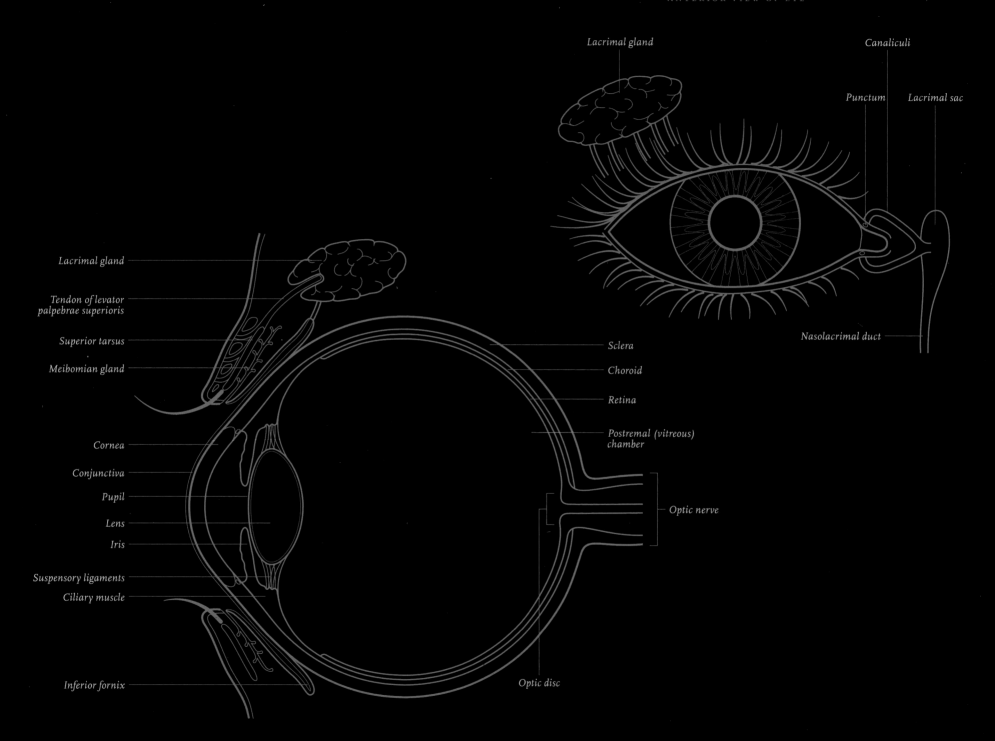

Lacrimal gland

Canaliculi

Punctum

Lacrimal sac

Lacrimal gland

Tendon of levator
palpebrae superioris

Superior tarsus

Meibomian gland

Sclera

Choroid

Retina

Postremal (vitreous)
chamber

Nasolacrimal duct

Cornea

Conjunctiva

Pupil

Lens

Iris

Suspensory ligaments

Ciliary muscle

Optic nerve

Inferior fornix

Optic disc

SAGITTAL VIEW OF EYEBALL

LATERAL VIEW OF RIGHT EYE

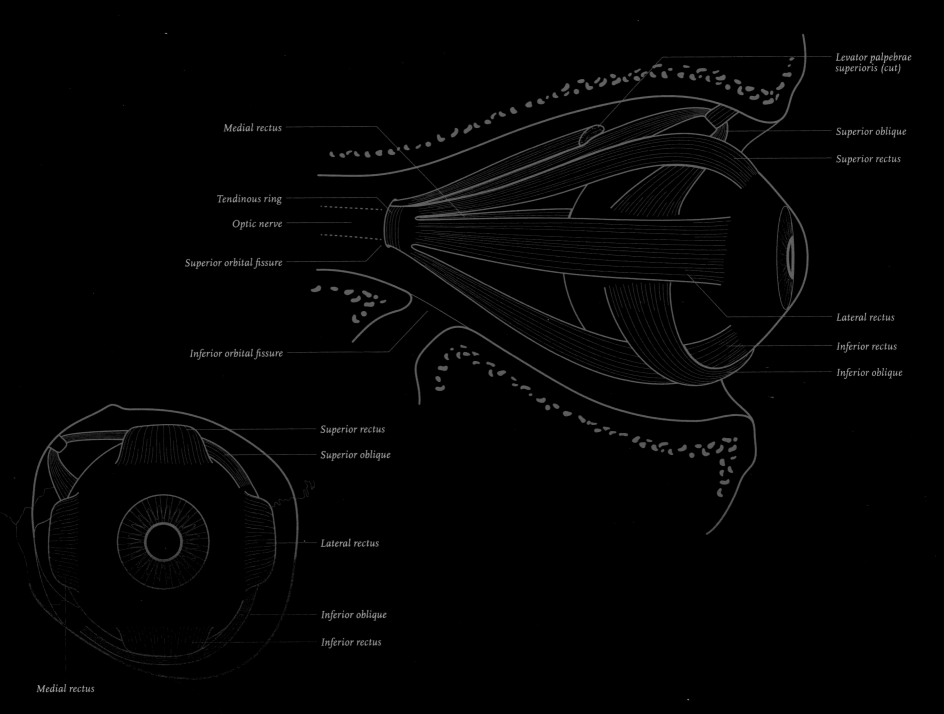

Levator palpebrae
superioris (cut)

Medial rectus

Superior oblique

Superior rectus

Tendinous ring

Optic nerve

Superior orbital fissure

Inferior orbital fissure

Lateral rectus

Inferior rectus

Inferior oblique

Superior rectus

Superior oblique

Lateral rectus

Inferior oblique

Inferior rectus

Medial rectus

VIEW OF ORBIT SHOWING NERVE SUPPLY TO EYE

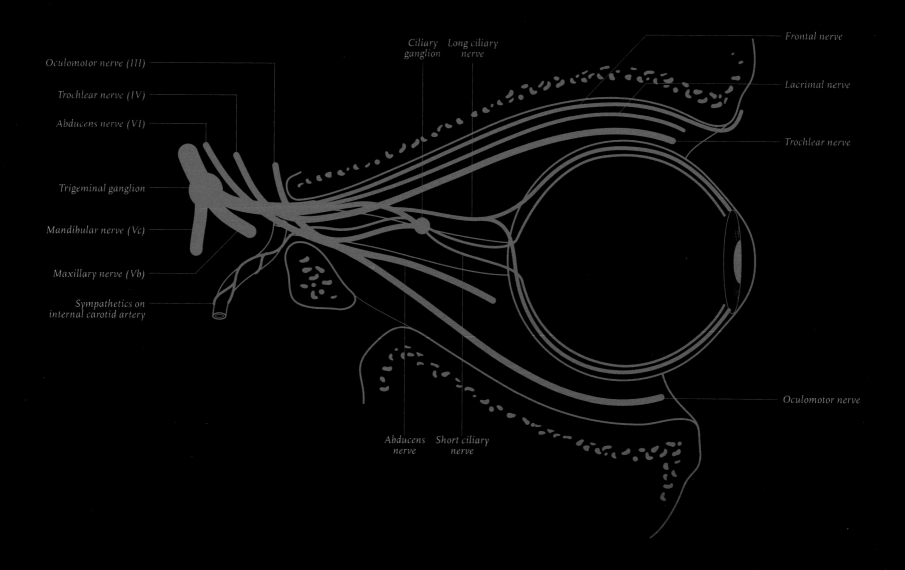

Oculomotor nerve (III)

Trochlear nerve (IV)

Abducens nerve (VI)

Trigeminal ganglion

Mandibular nerve (Vc)

Maxillary nerve (Vb)

Sympathetics on internal carotid artery

Ciliary ganglion

Long ciliary nerve

Frontal nerve

Lacrimal nerve

Trochlear nerve

Oculomotor nerve

Abducens nerve

Short ciliary nerve

HORIZONTAL SECTION THROUGH LEFT EYE

OPHTHALMOSCOPIC VIEW OF LEFT RETINA

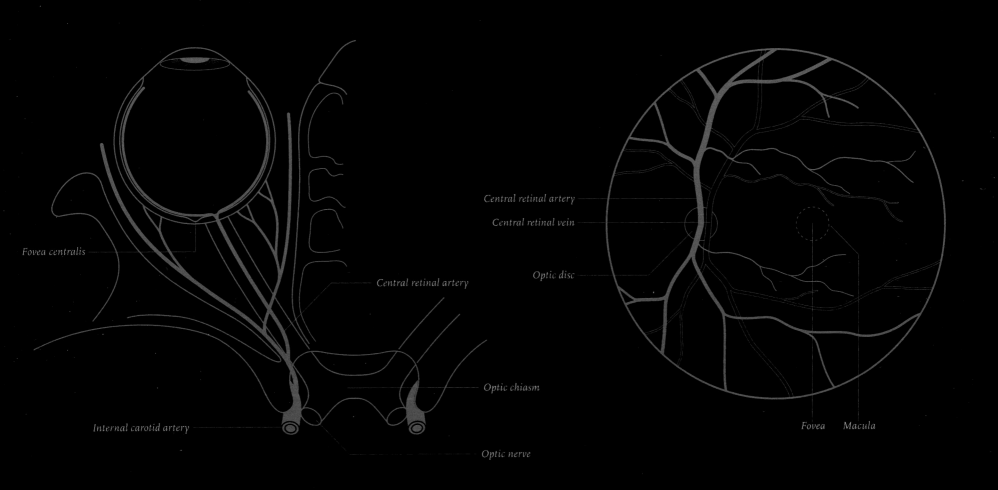

Fovea centralis

Central retinal artery

Optic chiasm

Internal carotid artery

Optic nerve

Central retinal artery

Central retinal vein

Optic disc

Fovea   *Macula*

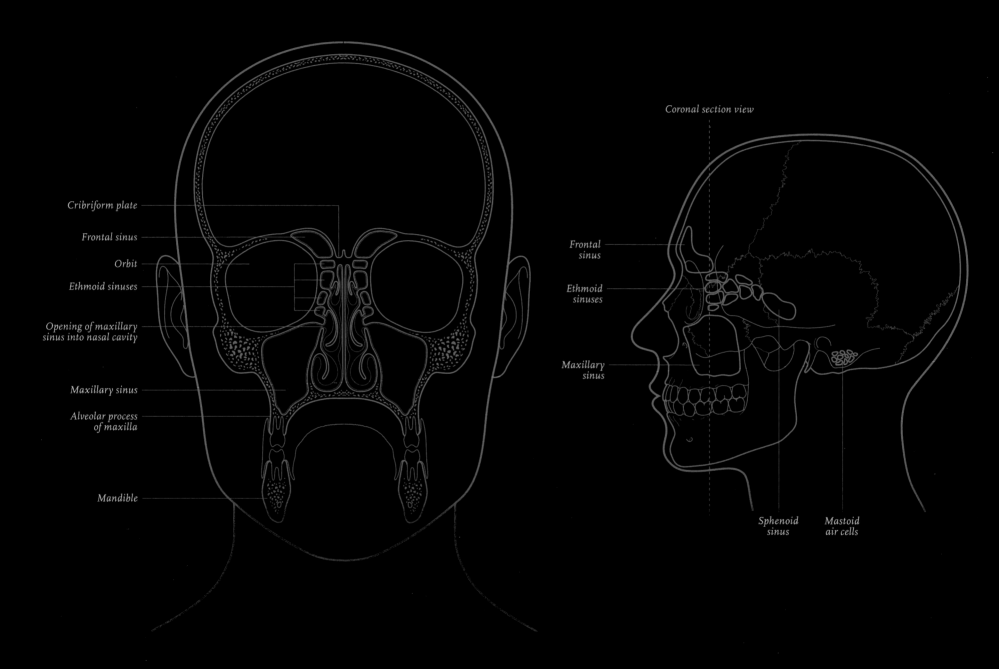

Cribriform plate

Frontal sinus

Orbit

Ethmoid sinuses

Opening of maxillary
sinus into nasal cavity

Maxillary sinus

Alveolar process
of maxilla

Mandible

Coronal section view

Frontal
sinus

Ethmoid
sinuses

Maxillary
sinus

Sphenoid
sinus

Mastoid
air cells

LATERAL VIEW OF NASAL CAVITY

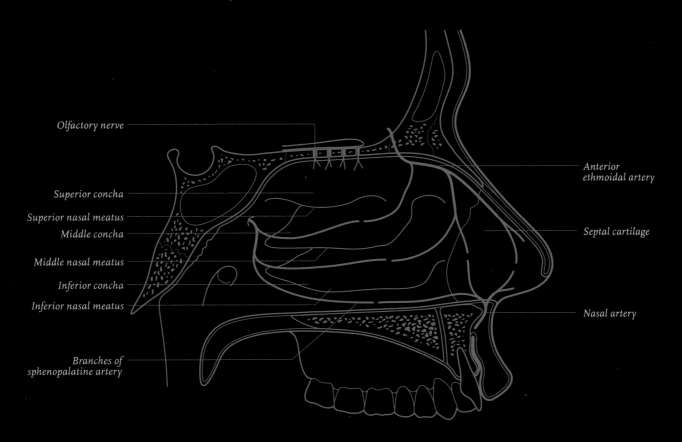

Olfactory nerve

Superior concha

Superior nasal meatus

Middle concha

Middle nasal meatus

Inferior concha

Inferior nasal meatus

Branches of
sphenopalatine artery

Anterior
ethmoidal artery

Septal cartilage

Nasal artery

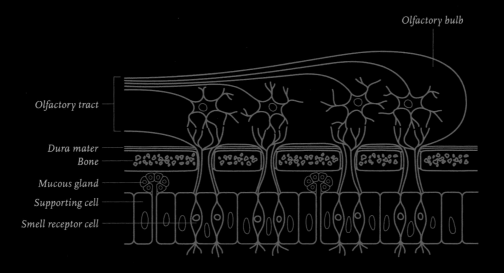

Olfactory bulb

Olfactory tract

Dura mater

Bone

Mucous gland

Supporting cell

Smell receptor cell

SAGITTAL VIEW OF OLFACTORY NERVE

CORONAL VIEW OF INNER EAR

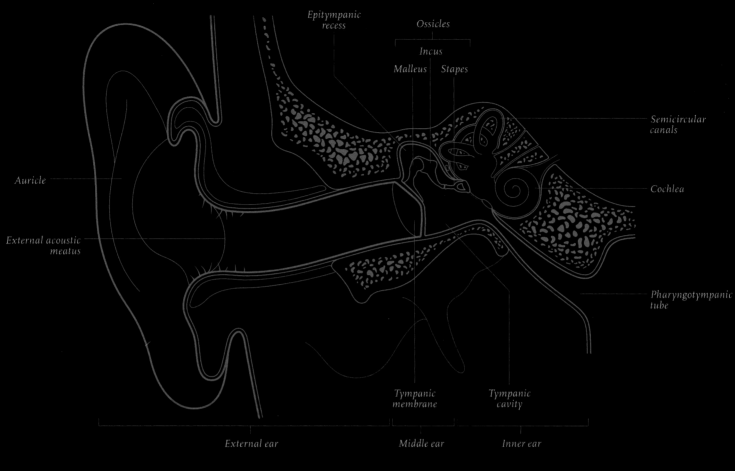

Epitympanic recess

Ossicles

Incus

Malleus | Stapes

Semicircular canals

Auricle

Cochlea

External acoustic meatus

Pharyngotympanic tube

Tympanic membrane

Tympanic cavity

External ear

Middle ear

Inner ear

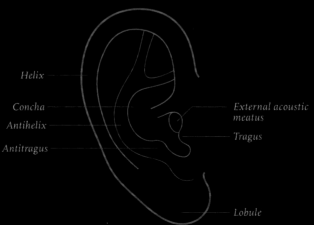

Helix

Concha

External acoustic meatus

Antihelix

Tragus

Antitragus

Lobule

LATERAL VIEW OF EXTERNAL EAR

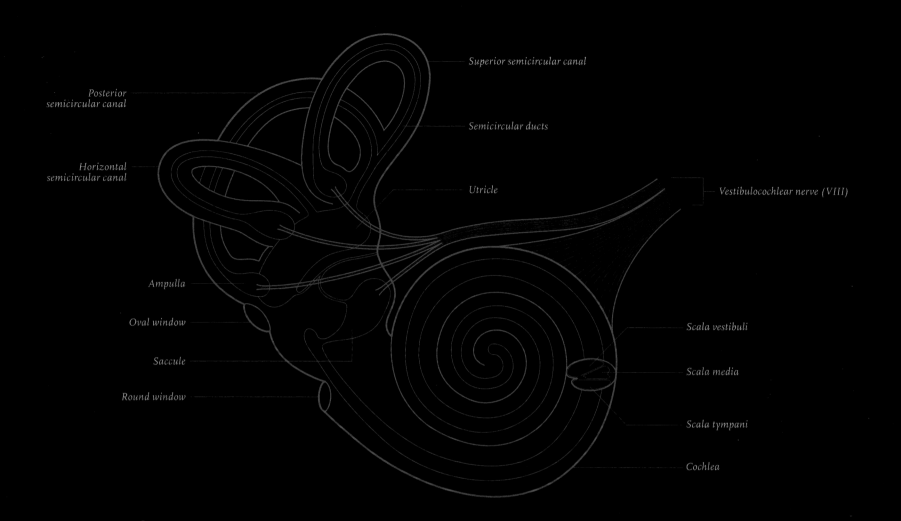

Superior semicircular canal

Posterior
semicircular canal

Semicircular ducts

Horizontal
semicircular canal

Utricle

Vestibulocochlear nerve (VIII)

Ampulla

Oval window

Scala vestibuli

Saccule

Scala media

Round window

Scala tympani

Cochlea

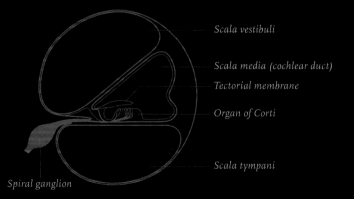

Scala vestibuli

Scala media (cochlear duct)

Tectorial membrane

Organ of Corti

Scala tympani

Spiral ganglion

SECTION THROUGH COCHLEA

THE NECK

The sternocleidomastoid muscle divides the neck into two regions: the anterior triangle and the posterior triangle. Working unilaterally, sternocleidomastoid tilts the head laterally on the same side while rotating the face in the opposite direction. Working bilaterally, they lift the chin upwards, extending the cervical vertebrae.

Boundaries of the posterior triangle are the anterior border of trapezius, the posterior border of sternocleidomastoid and the middle third of the clavicle. Within this triangle, the muscles arise from the skull and cervical vertebrae and insert into the ribs (scalenes), scapula (levator scapulae, omohyoid) and vertebral spines (splenius capitis, semispinalis capitis).

Boundaries of the anterior triangle are the anterior border of sternocleidomastoid, the inferior aspect of the mandible and the midline between the suprasternal notch and mandible.

The hyoid bone divides the muscles into suprahyoid and infrahyoid groups. The suprahyoid muscles elevate the hyoid bone and the floor of the mouth during swallowing, whereas the infrahyoids resist elevation of the hyoid bone during swallowing. Thyrohyoid and sternothyroid also elevate and depress the larynx respectively for aiding sound production.

Anterior to the bodies of the cervical vertebrae lies the pharynx, a tube formed by slings of constrictor muscles suspended from the pharyngeal tubercle at the base of the skull. They work sequentially to squeeze food from the oropharynx, at the back of the mouth, down to the oesophagus. A collection of palatine muscles assists the efficacy of the constrictors by elevating the soft palate during swallowing, thus blocking the nasopharynx and preventing food from entering the nasal cavity. Once the food bolus descends into the laryngopharynx, helped by the middle and inferior constrictors, it slides over the vallecular surface of the cartilaginous epiglottis to prevent it from entering the laryngeal inlet.

Condensations of lymphoid tissue (tubal tonsils, adenoids, palatine tonsils, lingual tonsils) surround the nasal and oral entrances to the pharynx, serving as a ring of immune protection.

The larynx is formed from a collection of cartilages and ligaments, which both assist in sound production whilst simultaneously preventing matter from entering the respiratory tract. Folds of mucosa-covered ligaments called vocal folds are stretched between the arytenoid and the thyroid cartilages. As air is passed through the space between the folds (rima glottidis), they can be moved into a position where they will vibrate, giving a sound. Swivel and sliding movements of the arytenoids on the cricoid cartilage open and close the cords, while movements between the thyroid and cricoid cartilages alter the pitch of the sound that is produced. With the exception of the cricothyroid muscle, which has its own branch of the vagus, the recurrent laryngeal nerve (branch of the vagus nerve, CN X) supplies all the intrinsic muscles of the larynx.

Surrounding the second to fourth tracheal cartilages inferior to the cricoid is the thyroid gland. Its function is to produce the hormone thyroxine, which controls basal metabolic rate. On the posterior surface of the thyroid gland lie four parathyroid glands, which secrete parathormone, controlling serum calcium levels. Blood supply of the thyroid is via superior and inferior thyroid arteries.

LATERAL VIEW OF SUPERFICIAL NECK MUSCLES

LATERAL VIEW OF DEEP NECK MUSCLES

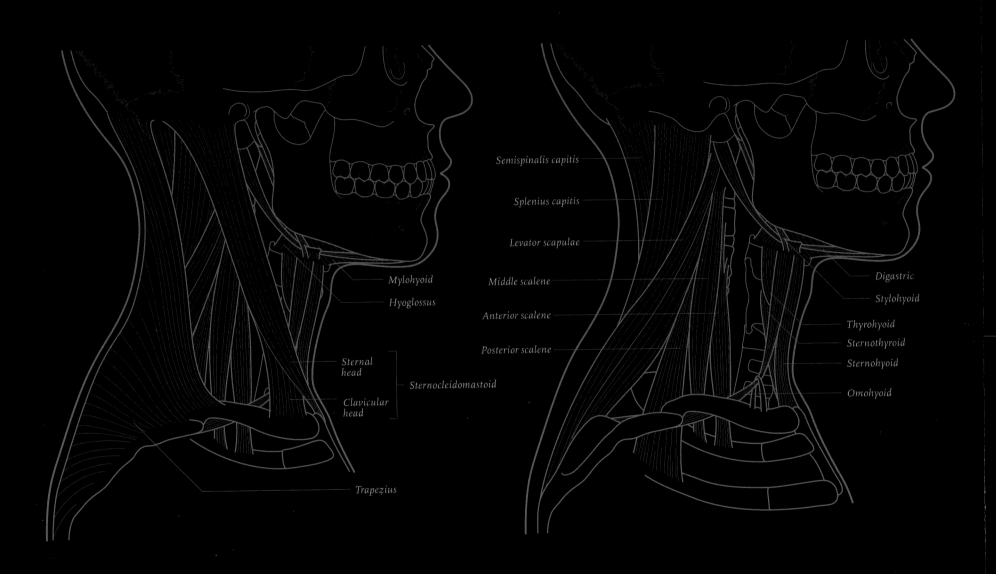

Mylohyoid

Hyoglossus

Sternal
head

Clavicular
head

Sternocleidomastoid

Trapezius

Semispinalis capitis

Splenius capitis

Levator scapulae

Middle scalene

Anterior scalene

Posterior scalene

Digastric

Stylohyoid

Thyrohyoid

Sternothyroid

Sternohyoid

Omohyoid

48

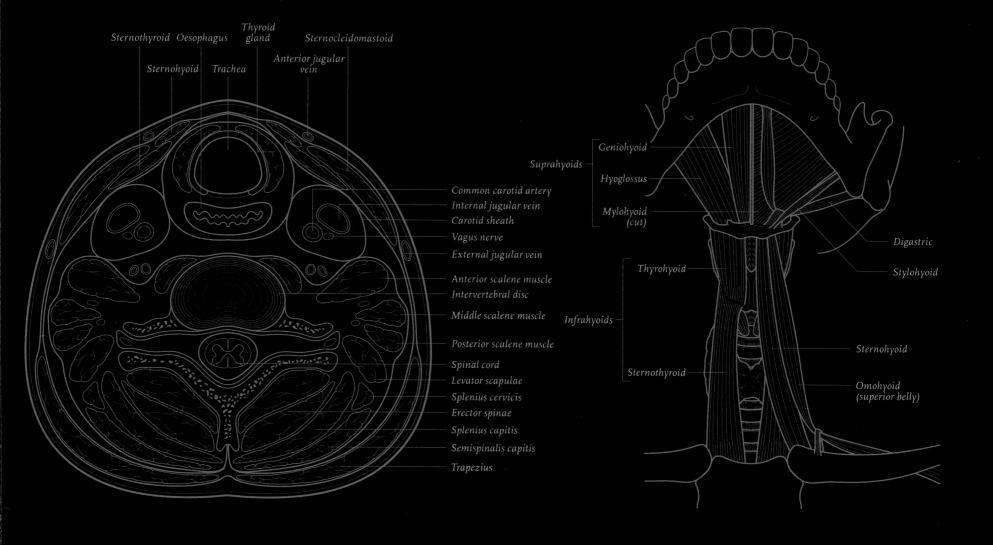

Sternothyroid Oesophagus

Thyroid
gland

Sternocleidomastoid

Sternohyoid   Trachea

Anterior jugular
vein

Common carotid artery
Internal jugular vein
Carotid sheath
Vagus nerve
External jugular vein

Anterior scalene muscle
Intervertebral disc

Middle scalene muscle

Posterior scalene muscle

Spinal cord
Levator scapulae
Splenius cervicis
Erector spinae
Splenius capitis
Semispinalis capitis
Trapezius

Suprahyoids

Geniohyoid

Hyoglossus

Mylohyoid
(cut)

Digastric

Stylohyoid

Thyrohyoid

Infrahyoids

Sternohyoid

Sternothyroid

Omohyoid
(superior belly)

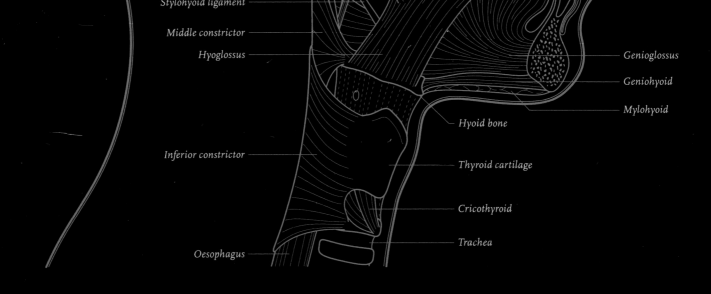

Stylohyoid ligament

Middle constrictor

Hyoglossus

Genioglossus

Geniohyoid

Mylohyoid

Hyoid bone

Inferior constrictor

Thyroid cartilage

Cricothyroid

Trachea

Oesophagus

POSTERIOR VIEW OF PHARYNX

INTERNAL VIEW OF PHARYNX

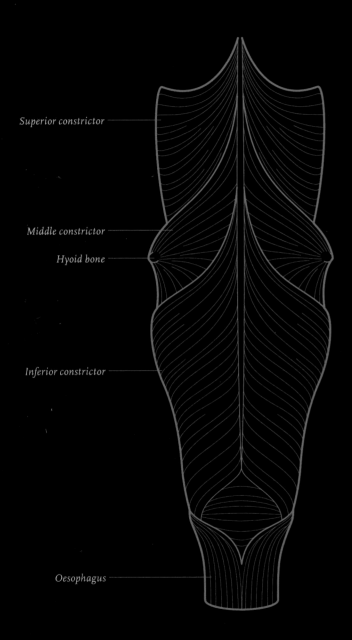

Superior constrictor

Middle constrictor

Hyoid bone

Inferior constrictor

Oesophagus

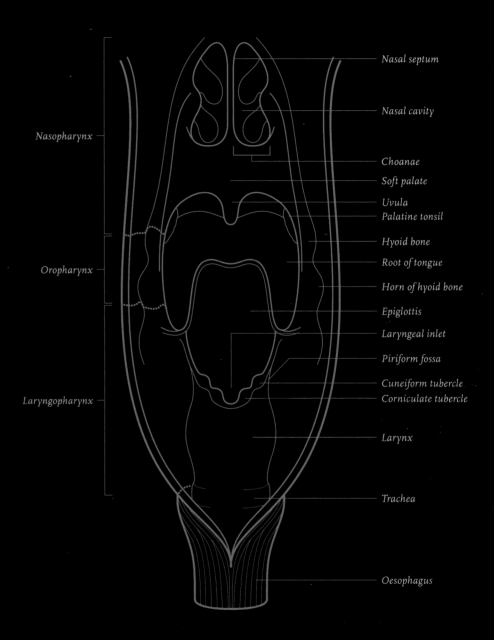

Nasopharynx

Oropharynx

Laryngopharynx

Nasal septum

Nasal cavity

Choanae

Soft palate

Uvula

Palatine tonsil

Hyoid bone

Root of tongue

Horn of hyoid bone

Epiglottis

Laryngeal inlet

Piriform fossa

Cuneiform tubercle

Corniculate tubercle

Larynx

Trachea

Oesophagus

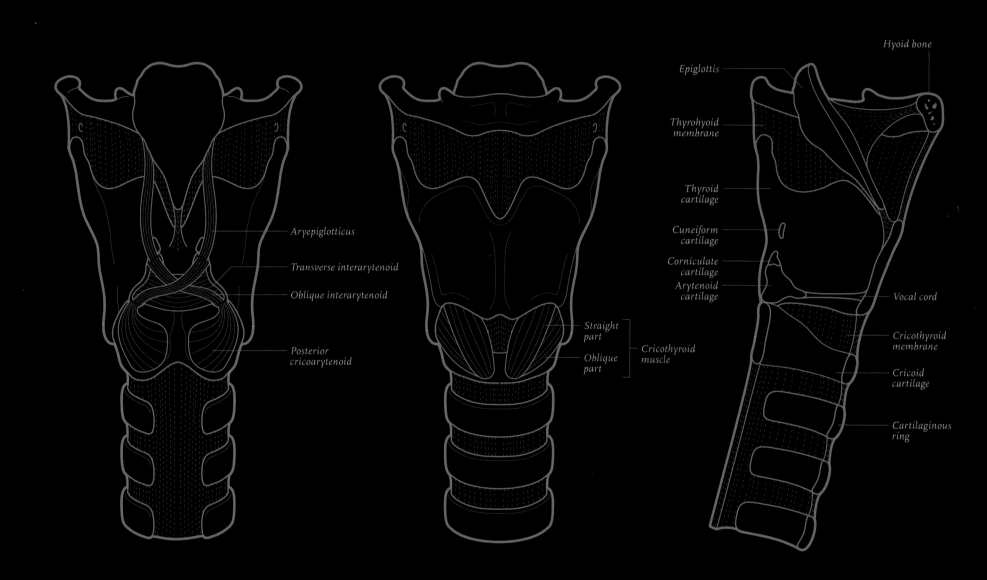

POSTERIOR VIEW OF LARYNX

ANTERIOR VIEW OF LARYNX

SAGITTAL VIEW OF LARYNX

Aryepiglotticus

Transverse interarytenoid

Oblique interarytenoid

Posterior
cricoarytenoid

Straight
part

Oblique
part

Cricothyroid
muscle

Epiglottis

Thyrohyoid
membrane

Thyroid
cartilage

Cuneiform
cartilage

Corniculate
cartilage

Arytenoid
cartilage

Hyoid bone

Vocal cord

Cricothyroid
membrane

Cricoid
cartilage

Cartilaginous
ring

SAGITTAL VIEW OF LARYNX

SUPERIOR VIEW OF LARYNX

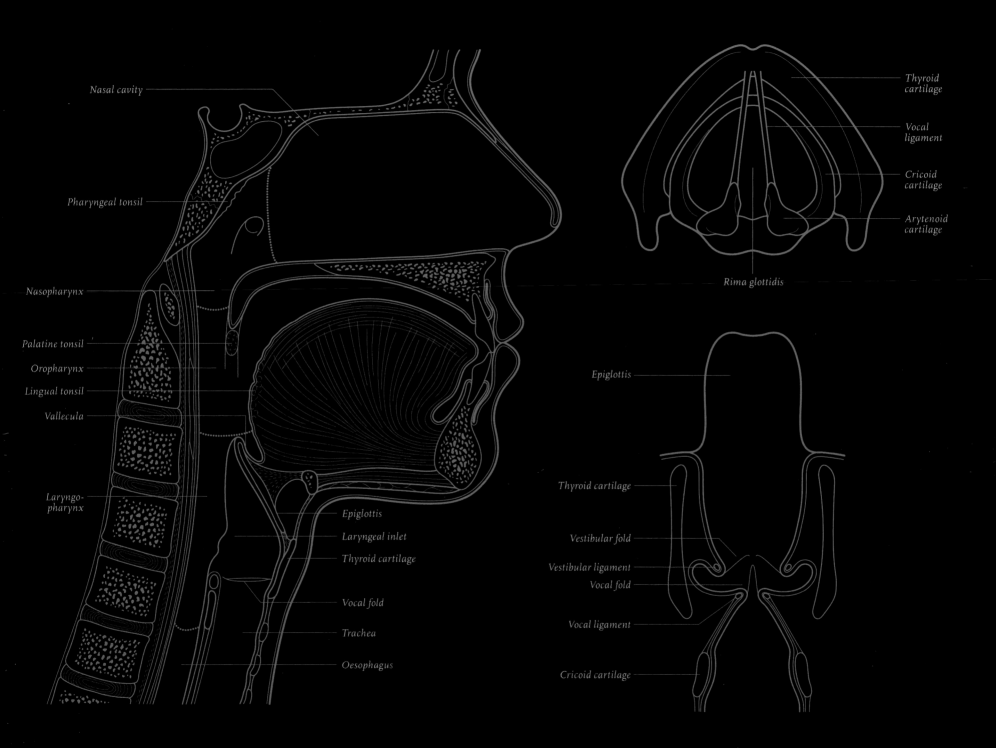

Nasal cavity

Pharyngeal tonsil

Nasopharynx

Palatine tonsil

Oropharynx

Lingual tonsil

Vallecula

Laryngo-
pharynx

Epiglottis

Laryngeal inlet

Thyroid cartilage

Vocal fold

Trachea

Oesophagus

Thyroid
cartilage

Vocal
ligament

Cricoid
cartilage

Arytenoid
cartilage

Rima glottidis

Epiglottis

Thyroid cartilage

Vestibular fold

Vestibular ligament

Vocal fold

Vocal ligament

Cricoid cartilage

CORONAL VIEW OF LARYNX

ANTERIOR VIEW OF THYROID GLAND

POSTERIOR VIEW OF THYROID GLAND

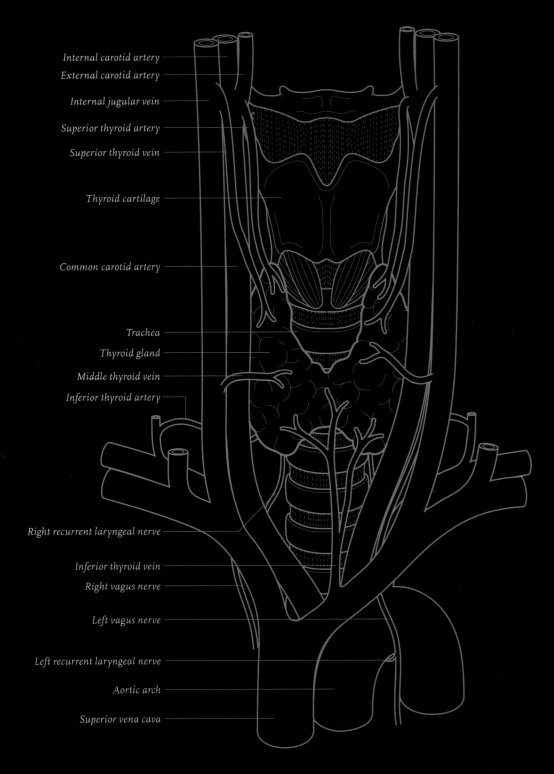

Internal carotid artery
External carotid artery
Internal jugular vein
Superior thyroid artery
Superior thyroid vein

Thyroid cartilage

Common carotid artery

Trachea
Thyroid gland
Middle thyroid vein
Inferior thyroid artery

Right recurrent laryngeal nerve

Inferior thyroid vein
Right vagus nerve

Left vagus nerve

Left recurrent laryngeal nerve

Aortic arch

Superior vena cava

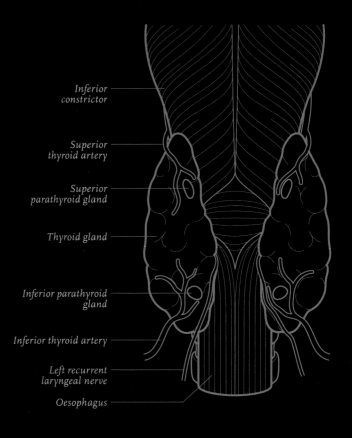

Inferior
constrictor

Superior
thyroid artery

Superior
parathyroid gland

Thyroid gland

Inferior parathyroid
gland

Inferior thyroid artery

Left recurrent
laryngeal nerve

Oesophagus

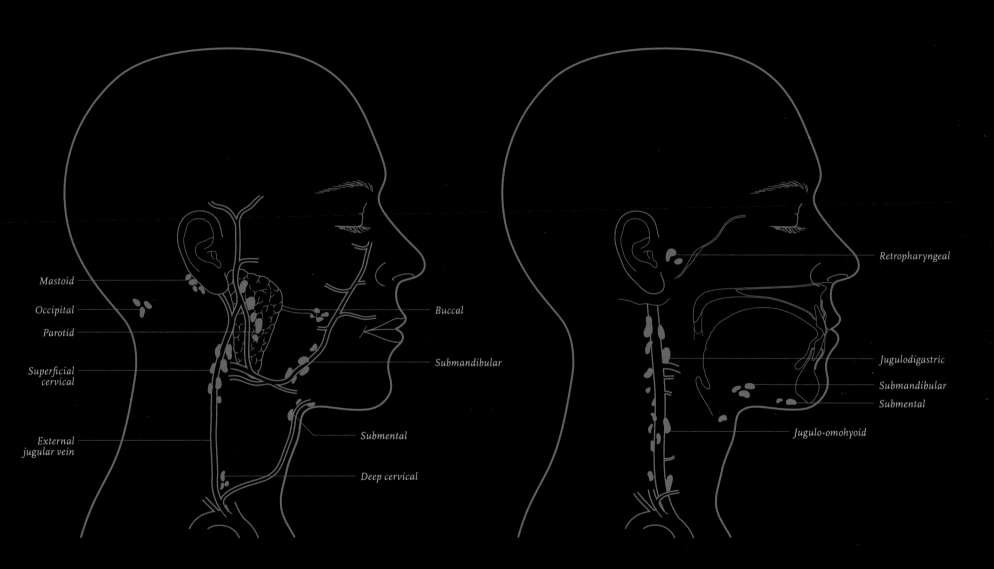

Mastoid

Occipital

Parotid

Superficial
cervical

External
jugular vein

Buccal

Submandibular

Submental

Deep cervical

Retropharyngeal

Jugulodigastric

Submandibular

Submental

Jugulo-omohyoid

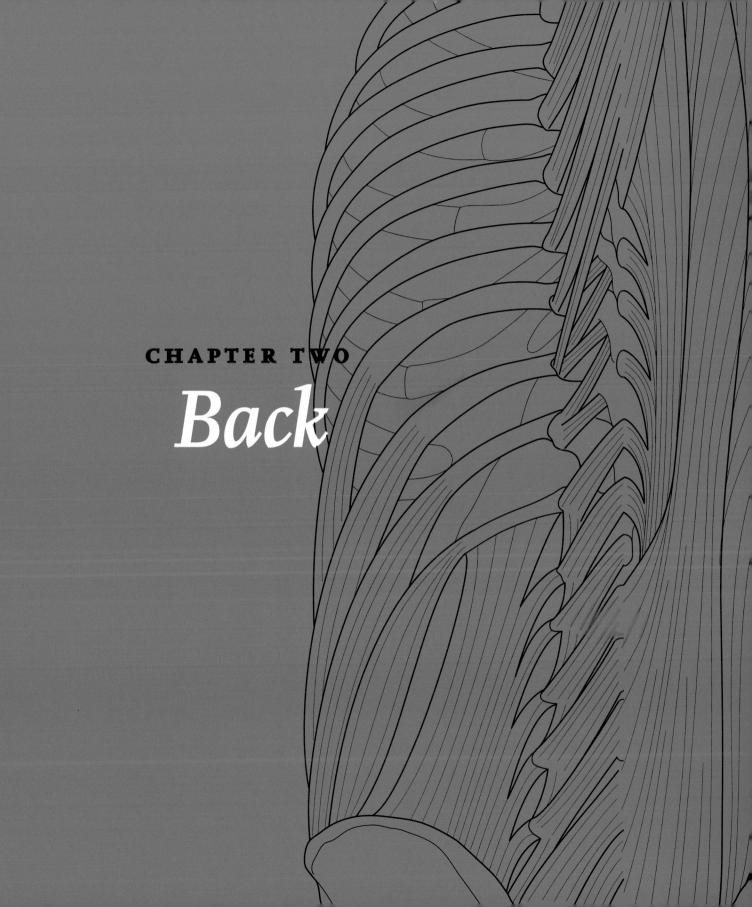

CHAPTER TWO
Back

support the weight of the trunk, carry the head and transmit forces to the lower limbs through the pelvis. The vertebrae are connected by muscles and ligaments to the skull, ribs and pelvis.

There are 24 true vertebrae, plus the sacrum and coccyx. The true vertebrae are segregated into categories: 7 cervical, 12 thoracic and 5 lumbar. The 5 sacral vertebrae are fused, as are the 4 coccygeal vertebrae. The thoracic and sacral regions maintain their embryonic primary curvature, whilst the cervical and lumbar secondary curvatures reflect the development of postural reflexes and onset of walking respectively.

The vertebrae articulate with one another through three joints. Anteriorly, an intervertebral disc lies between the vertebral bodies and, posteriorly, two synovial facet joints lie between the superior and inferior articular processes.

called the anulus fibrosus surround the central watery nucleus pulposus of the intervertebral disc. This allows partial movement between vertebral bodies. All joints are secured by strong ligaments to keep the spinal movements stable, with the greatest amount of movement achievable by the cervical spine.

Shapes of the vertebrae vary depending on where they are located along the length of the vertebral column. Their relative shape is determined by a number of factors such as their weight-bearing ability, giving a large vertebral body in the lumbar vertebrae, or if they articulate with the ribs via facets on the thoracic vertebrae.

Posterior to the vertebral body is the vertebral canal. This carries the spinal cord, which originates at the foramen magnum of the skull as an extension of the brain. Vertebral foramina between articulated vertebrae transmit the spinal nerves to their destinations within the body.

are continuous with those of the brain; thus the cord is also bathed in CSF. At around the level of L1, the spinal cord terminates at the conus medullaris, and the cauda equina (horse's tail) is its continuation as the lumbar, sacral and coccygeal nerve roots in the subarachnoid space.

The muscular architecture of the back can be divided into extrinsic muscles (those concerned with moving the upper limbs and thoracic wall) and intrinsic muscles (those maintaining posture and allowing movements such as flexion, extension, lateral flexion and rotation of the vertebral column). The intrinsic muscles can be classified as those innervated by the posterior rami of spinal nerves, and are noted as the erector spinae, splenius, suboccipital and transversospinalis muscle groups.

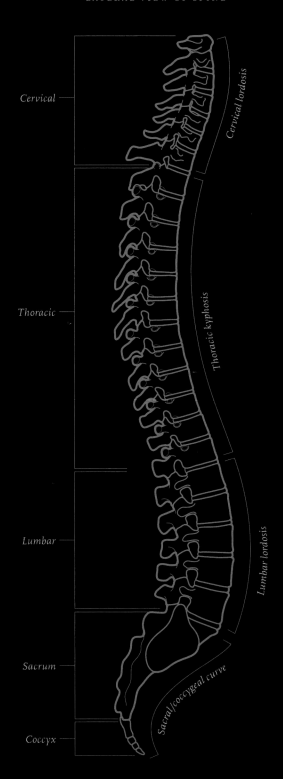

Cervical

Cervical lordosis

Thoracic

Thoracic kyphosis

Lumbar

Lumbar lordosis

Sacrum

Sacral/coccygeal curve

Coccyx

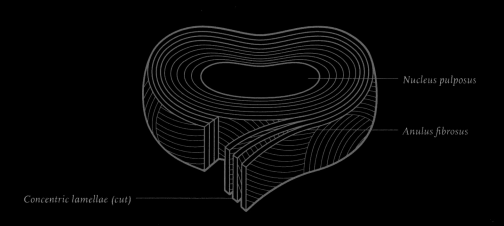

Nucleus pulposus

Anulus fibrosus

Concentric lamellae (cut)

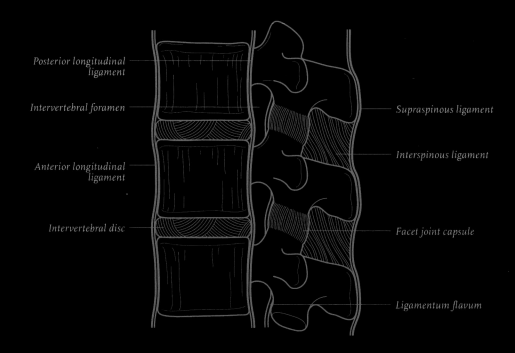

Posterior longitudinal ligament

Intervertebral foramen

Anterior longitudinal ligament

Intervertebral disc

Supraspinous ligament

Interspinous ligament

Facet joint capsule

Ligamentum flavum

LATERAL VIEW OF SPINAL MOTION SEGMENTS

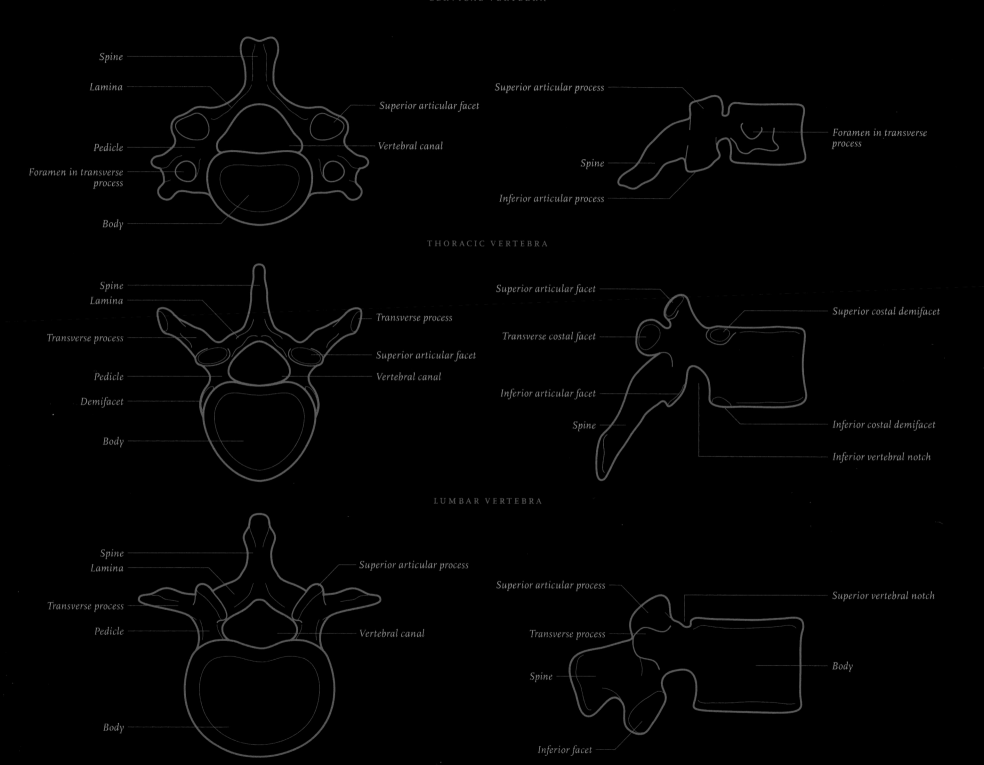

CERVICAL VERTEBRA

Spine

Lamina

Superior articular facet

Pedicle

Vertebral canal

Foramen in transverse
process

Body

Superior articular process

Foramen in transverse
process

Spine

Inferior articular process

THORACIC VERTEBRA

Spine
Lamina

Transverse process

Transverse process

Superior articular facet

Pedicle

Vertebral canal

Demifacet

Body

Superior articular facet

Superior costal demifacet

Transverse costal facet

Inferior articular facet

Spine

Inferior costal demifacet

Inferior vertebral notch

LUMBAR VERTEBRA

Spine
Lamina

Superior articular process

Transverse process

Pedicle

Vertebral canal

Body

Superior articular process

Superior vertebral notch

Transverse process

Spine

Body

Inferior facet

SAGITTAL VIEW THROUGH SPINE

SAGITTAL VIEW OF LUMBAR SPINE

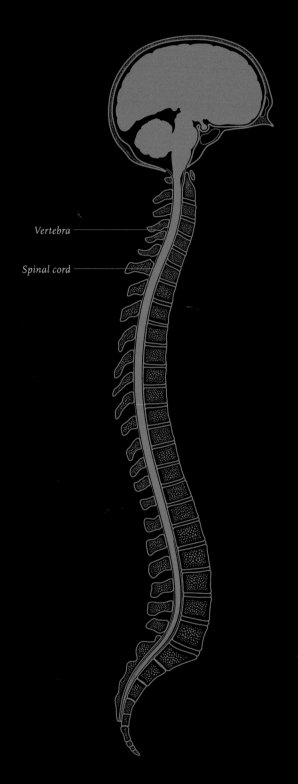

Vertebra

Spinal cord

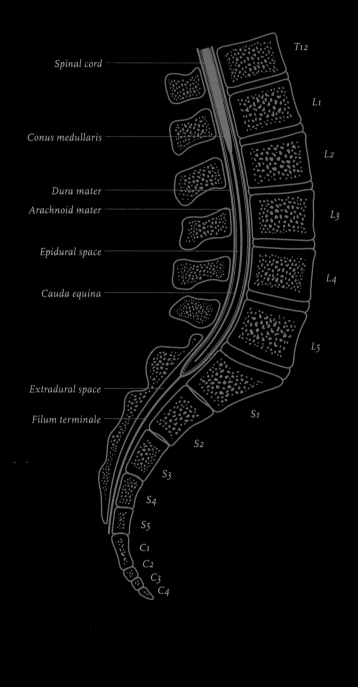

Spinal cord

Conus medullaris

Dura mater

Arachnoid mater

Epidural space

Cauda equina

Extradural space

Filum terminale

T12

L1

L2

L3

L4

L5

S1

S2

S3

S4

S5

C1

C2

C3

C4

TRANSVERSE SECTION OF THORACIC VERTEBRA WITH SPINAL CORD

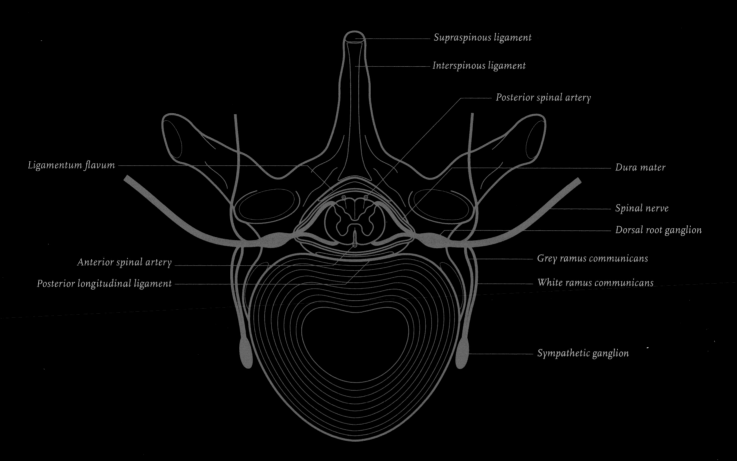

Supraspinous ligament

Interspinous ligament

Posterior spinal artery

Ligamentum flavum

Dura mater

Spinal nerve

Dorsal root ganglion

Anterior spinal artery

Grey ramus communicans

Posterior longitudinal ligament

White ramus communicans

Sympathetic ganglion

Posterior median sulcus

Posterior horn   White matter   Dorsal root

Anterior
horn

Grey
matter

Ventral
root

Anterior median fissure

TRANSVERSE SECTION THROUGH SPINAL CORD

POSTERIOR VIEW OF EXTRINSIC BACK MUSCLES

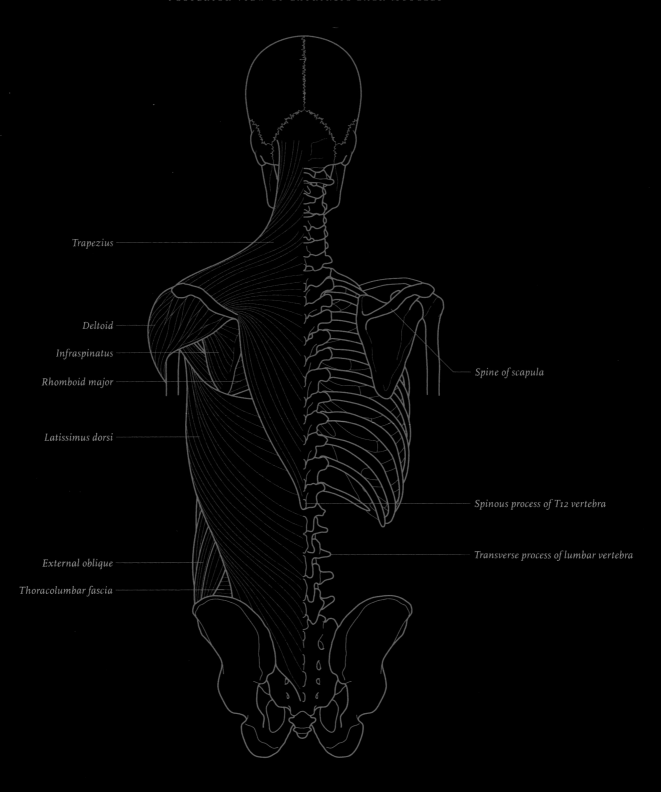

Trapezius

Deltoid

Infraspinatus

Rhomboid major

Latissimus dorsi

External oblique

Thoracolumbar fascia

Spine of scapula

Spinous process of T12 vertebra

Transverse process of lumbar vertebra

POSTERIOR VIEW OF INTRINSIC BACK MUSCLES

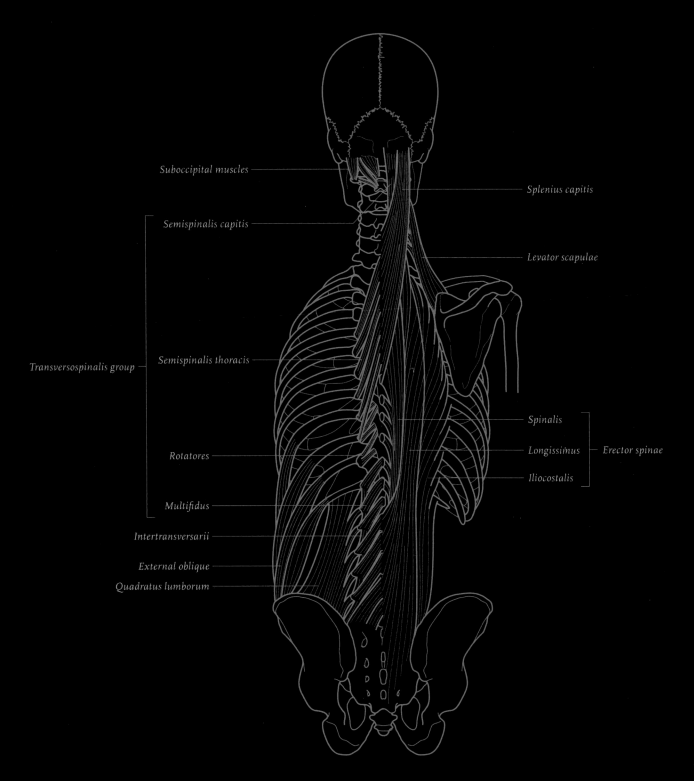

Suboccipital muscles

Splenius capitis

Semispinalis capitis

Levator scapulae

Transversospinalis group

Semispinalis thoracis

Spinalis

Longissimus — Erector spinae

Rotatores

Iliocostalis

Multifidus

Intertransversarii

External oblique

Quadratus lumborum

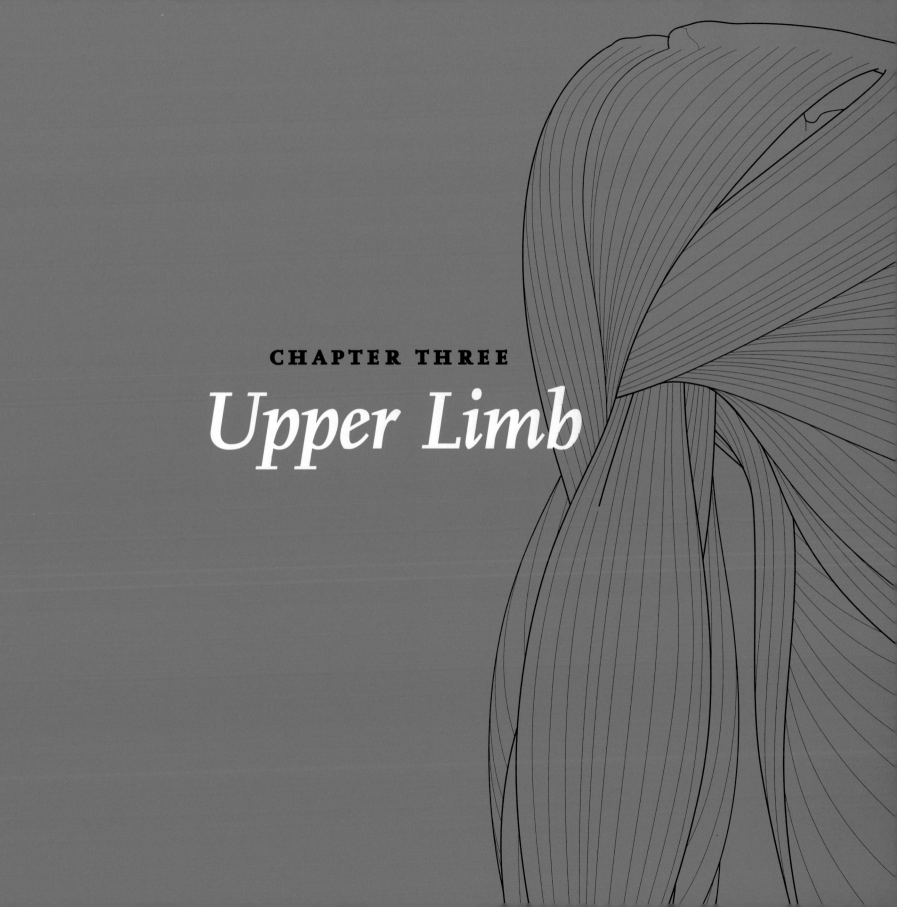

CHAPTER THREE
Upper Limb

Upper Limb

THE BONES & JOINTS

The upper limb is highly mobile to allow comprehensive positioning of the hand. This mobility is due to the arrangement of the pectoral girdle, comprising the clavicle and scapula. The only articulation of the upper limb to the axial skeleton is via the small synovial sternoclavicular joint between the clavicle and the sternum. The remainder of the pectoral girdle is a physiological attachment via muscles to the posterior thoracic wall. The 'S'-shaped clavicle articulates with the scapula at the synovial acromioclavicular joint and is reinforced by accessory acromioclavicular and coracoclavicular ligaments.

The shallow articular surface of the glenoid cavity of the scapula where the head of the humerus forms a synovial ball-and-socket joint is a true reflection of how stability has been sacrificed for mobility in the non-weight-bearing upper limb.

The glenoid cavity is deepened by the glenoid labrum, a fibrocartilaginous collar, and enveloped in a lax articular capsule strengthened by various glenohumeral ligaments.

The presence of two bones in the forearm means that there are three joints at the elbow: the humeroulnar joint between the ulna and the trochlea of the humerus, the radiohumeral joint between the head of the radius and the capitulum of the humerus, and the proximal radioulnar joint. All three joints are encapsulated in the same joint capsule. Although flexion and extension occur at the elbow, the radius can pivot around a stabilised ulna to facilitate supination (palm up) and pronation (palm down) movements.

There are eight wrist bones, of which three articulate with the distal radius and articular disc (scaphoid, lunate and triquetrum) forming the wrist joint. This joint allows flexion, extension, abduction and adduction of the hand. Radial and ulnar collateral ligaments reinforce the joint capsule. Movement at the synovial intercarpal joints is limited, but they still contribute to the positioning of the hand.

The most mobile of the carpometacarpal joints is the synovial saddle joint between the first metacarpal and trapezium, allowing for flexion, extension, abduction, adduction, rotation (opposition) and circumduction of the thumb.

Although both the proximal and distal interphalangeal hinge joint movements of the fingers are limited to flexion and extension, the condylar metacarpophalangeal joints allow the additional movements of abduction, adduction and circumduction.

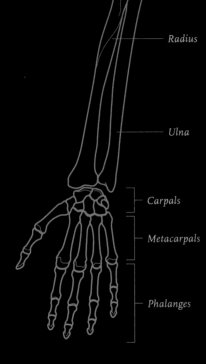

Radius

Ulna

Carpals

Metacarpals

Phalanges

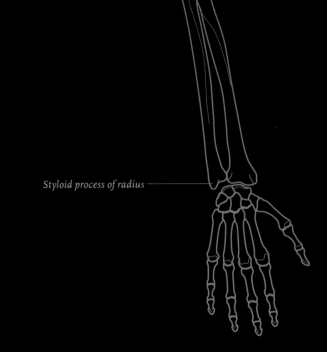

Styloid process of radius

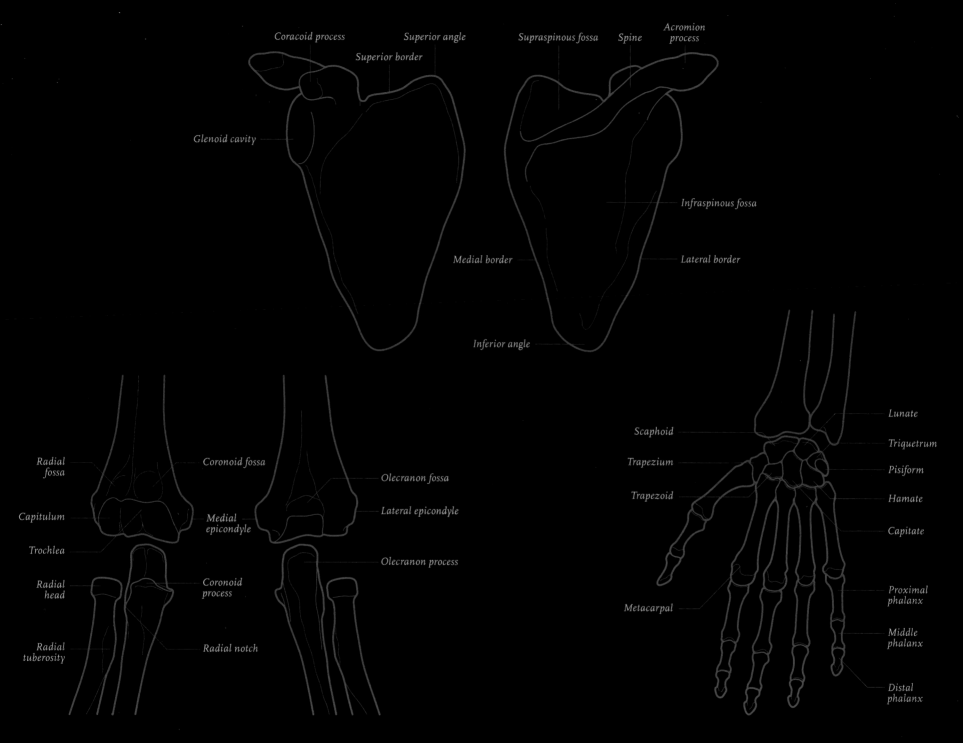

ANTERIOR VIEW OF SCAPULA

POSTERIOR VIEW OF SCAPULA

Coracoid process

Superior angle

Superior border

Supraspinous fossa

Spine

Acromion process

Glenoid cavity

Infraspinous fossa

Medial border

Lateral border

Inferior angle

Radial fossa

Coronoid fossa

Olecranon fossa

Capitulum

Medial epicondyle

Lateral epicondyle

Trochlea

Olecranon process

Radial head

Coronoid process

Radial tuberosity

Radial notch

Scaphoid

Lunate

Triquetrum

Trapezium

Pisiform

Trapezoid

Hamate

Capitate

Metacarpal

Proximal phalanx

Middle phalanx

Distal phalanx

ANTERIOR VIEW OF ELBOW

POSTERIOR VIEW OF ELBOW

PALMAR VIEW OF HAND

JOINTS OF PECTORAL GIRDLE & SHOULDER

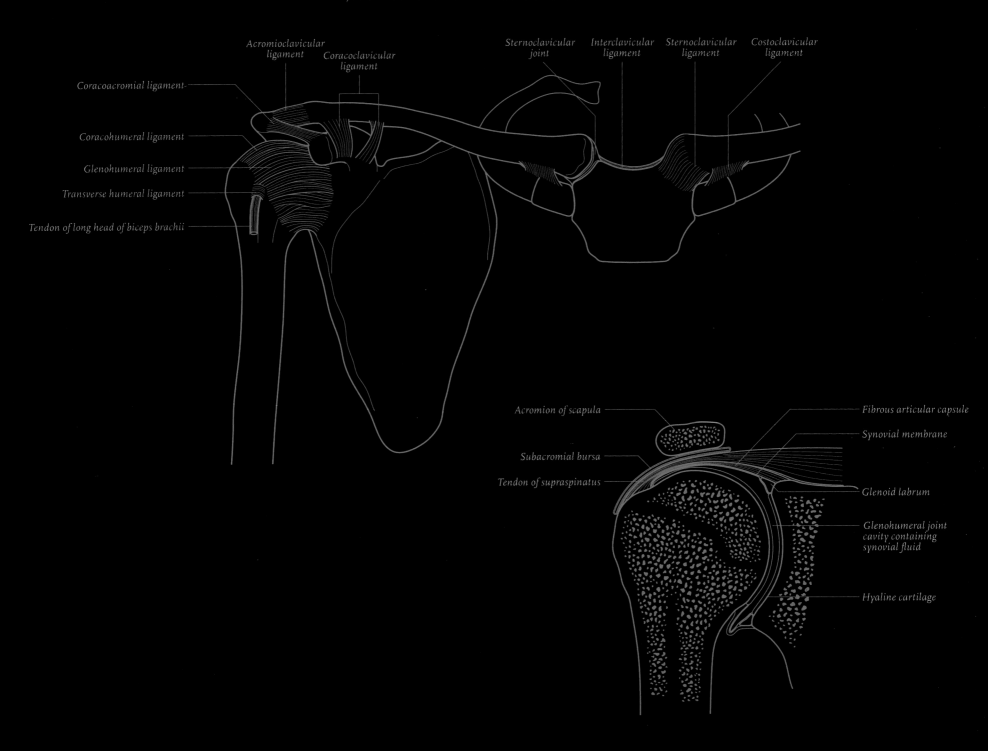

Acromioclavicular
ligament

Coracoclavicular
ligament

Coracoacromial ligament

Coracohumeral ligament

Glenohumeral ligament

Transverse humeral ligament

Tendon of long head of biceps brachii

Sternoclavicular
joint

Interclavicular
ligament

Sternoclavicular
ligament

Costoclavicular
ligament

Acromion of scapula

Subacromial bursa

Tendon of supraspinatus

Fibrous articular capsule

Synovial membrane

Glenoid labrum

Glenohumeral joint
cavity containing
synovial fluid

Hyaline cartilage

SECTION THROUGH GLENOHUMERAL JOINT

SAGITTAL VIEW OF ELBOW JOINT

SECTION THROUGH WRIST & HAND

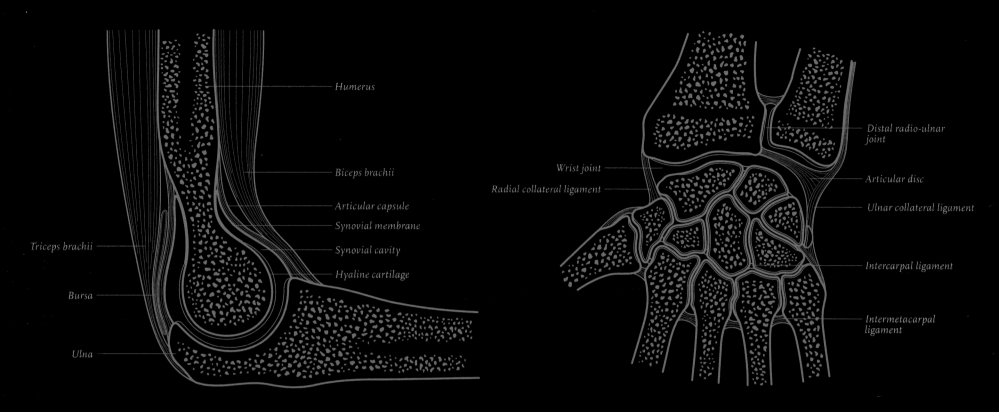

Humerus

Biceps brachii

Articular capsule

Synovial membrane

Synovial cavity

Hyaline cartilage

Triceps brachii

Bursa

Ulna

Distal radio-ulnar joint

Wrist joint

Radial collateral ligament

Articular disc

Ulnar collateral ligament

Intercarpal ligament

Intermetacarpal ligament

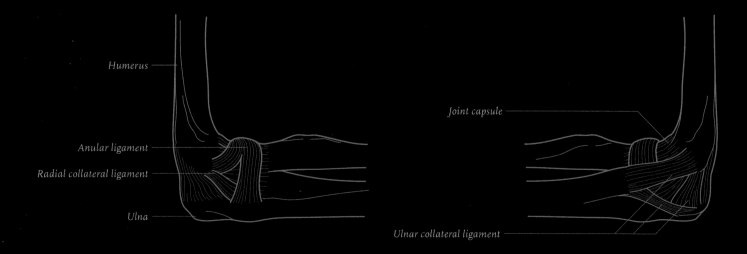

Humerus

Anular ligament

Radial collateral ligament

Ulna

Joint capsule

Ulnar collateral ligament

LATERAL VIEW OF ELBOW

MEDIAL VIEW OF ELBOW

The remainder of the muscles acting on the shoulder joint are numerous. Due to the multipennate structure of the deltoid muscle and its broad clavicular and scapular origin, different portions of it contribute to all the available movements: flexion, extension, abduction, adduction, and medial and lateral rotation.

Pectoralis major also facilitates a number of movements: its upper fibres flex the arm whilst its lower fibres extend the flexed joint. Teres major and pectoralis major both medially rotate the arm alongside latissimus dorsi, which is also

scapula and humerus and an insertion at the olecranon of the ulna, it is a powerful extensor. Anconeus assists triceps in this role.

The anterior compartment of the forearm is where the muscle bellies of the forearm flexors lie. Some arise from the medial epicondyle, flexing the wrist (flexor carpi radialis, flexor carpi ulnaris and palmaris longus). Others arise principally from the forearm bones and have tendons that travel through the carpal tunnel and insert into the phalanges of the digits. Flexor digitorum superficialis (FDS) flexes the proximal interphalangeal joints, whilst the tendons of

Some of these arise from the tendons of FDP and are termed the lumbricals, which, together with the interossei, insert into the extensor expansion, allowing flexion of the metacarpophalangeal joints and extension of the interphalangeal joints. Additionally, the interossei adduct (palmar interossei) and abduct (dorsal interossei) the metacarpals.

The muscles of the thenar eminence and hypothenar eminence coordinate a range of possible movements, including opposition of the thumb and little finger to one another.

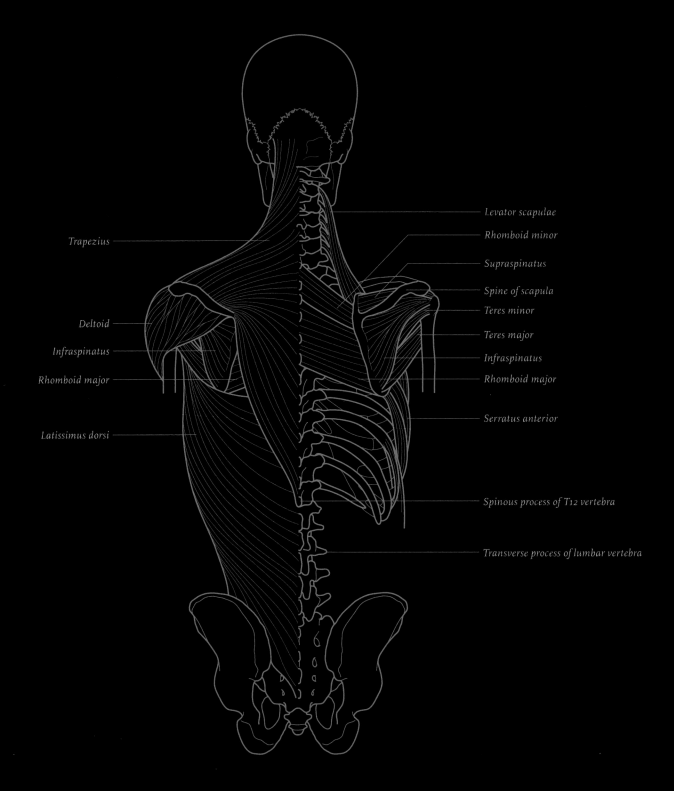

Levator scapulae

Rhomboid minor

Supraspinatus

Spine of scapula

Teres minor

Teres major

Infraspinatus

Rhomboid major

Serratus anterior

Spinous process of T12 vertebra

Transverse process of lumbar vertebra

Trapezius

Deltoid

Infraspinatus

Rhomboid major

Latissimus dorsi

ANTERIOR VIEW OF SHOULDER MUSCLES

POSTERIOR VIEW OF SCAPULAR MUSCLES

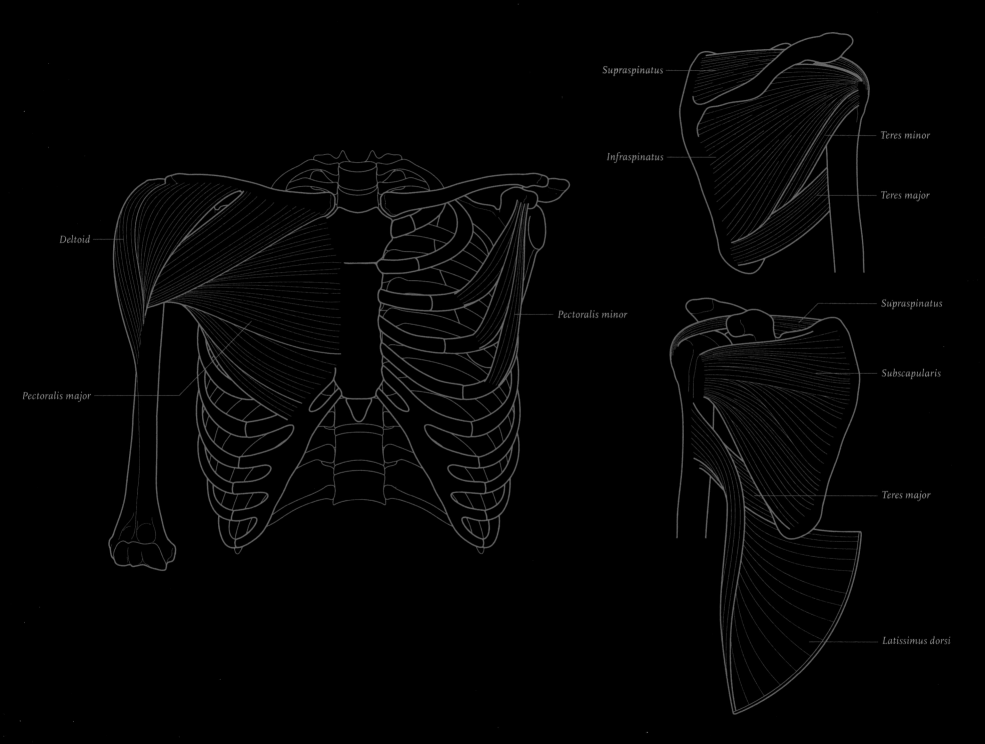

Supraspinatus

Infraspinatus

Teres minor

Teres major

Deltoid

Supraspinatus

Pectoralis minor

Subscapularis

Pectoralis major

Teres major

Latissimus dorsi

ANTERIOR VIEW OF SHOULDER MUSCLES

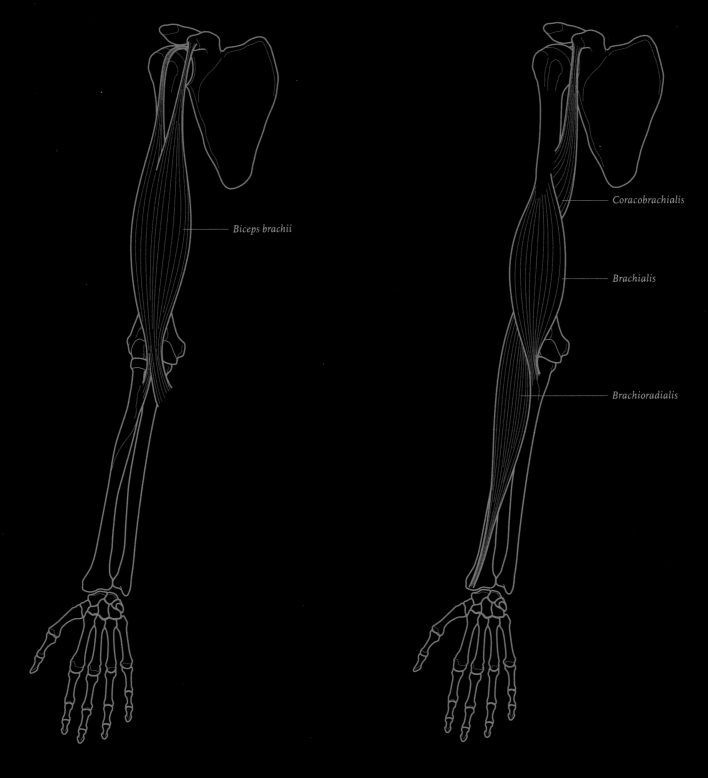

Biceps brachii

Coracobrachialis

Brachialis

Brachioradialis

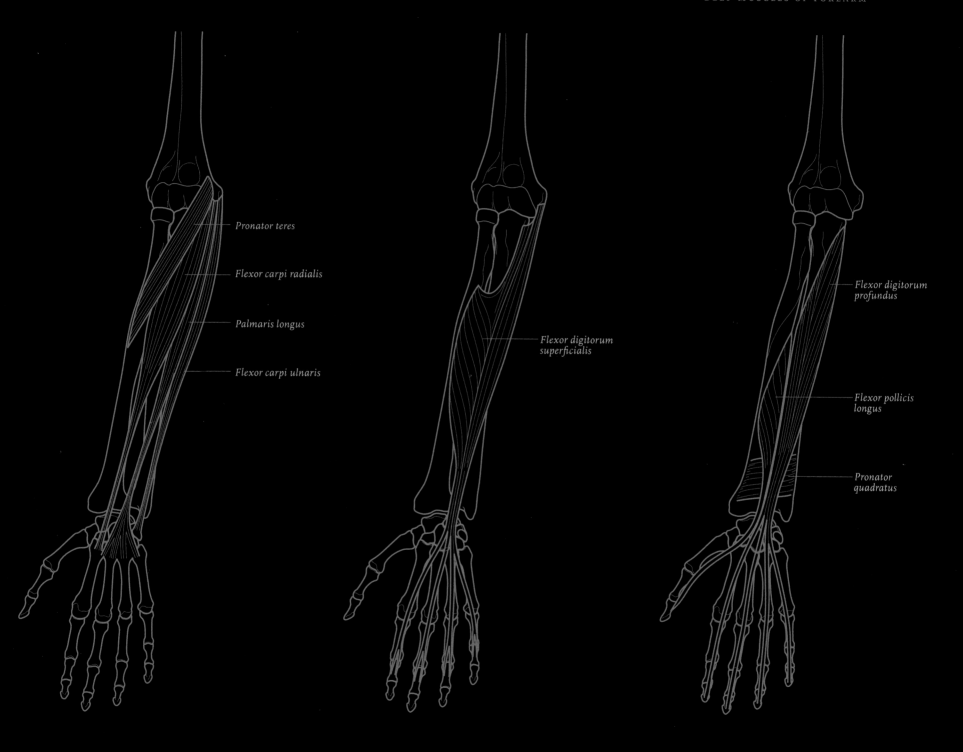

ANTERIOR VIEW OF
SUPERFICIAL MUSCLES OF FOREARM

ANTERIOR VIEW OF
INTERMEDIATE MUSCLE OF FOREARM

ANTERIOR VIEW OF
DEEP MUSCLES OF FOREARM

Pronator teres

Flexor carpi radialis

Palmaris longus

Flexor carpi ulnaris

Flexor digitorum superficialis

Flexor digitorum profundus

Flexor pollicis longus

Pronator quadratus

TRANSVERSE SECTION THROUGH ARM

POSTERIOR VIEW OF ARM MUSCLES

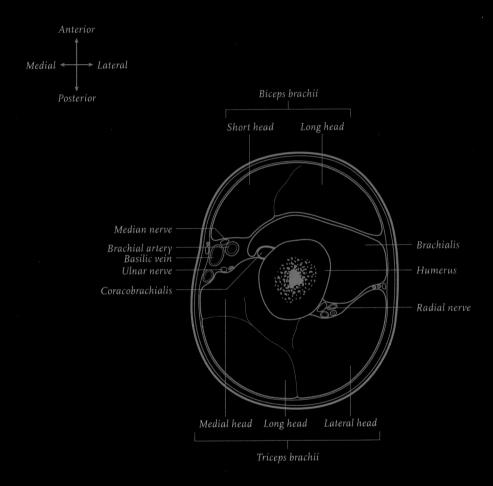

Anterior

Medial ← → *Lateral*

Posterior

Biceps brachii

Short head   Long head

Median nerve

Brachial artery

Basilic vein

Ulnar nerve

Coracobrachialis

Brachialis

Humerus

Radial nerve

Medial head   Long head   Lateral head

Triceps brachii

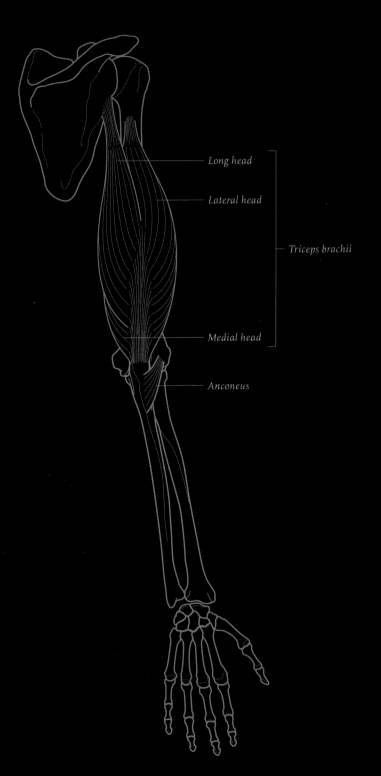

Long head

Lateral head

Triceps brachii

Medial head

Anconeus

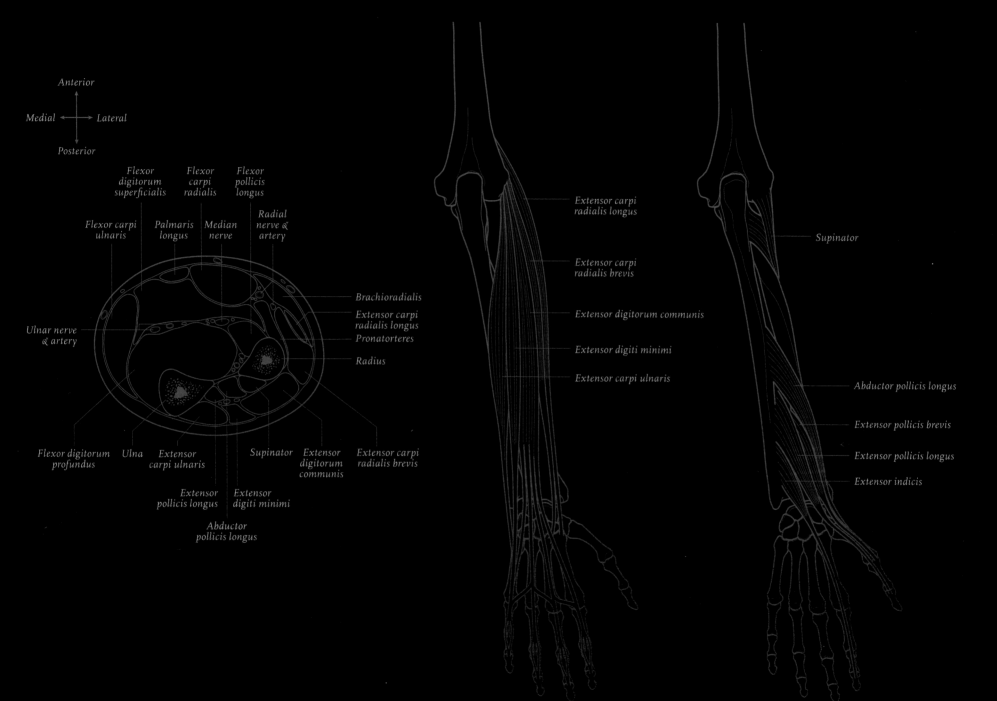

Anterior

Medial ←→ Lateral

Posterior

Flexor digitorum superficialis

Flexor carpi radialis

Flexor pollicis longus

Flexor carpi ulnaris

Palmaris longus

Median nerve

Radial nerve & artery

Ulnar nerve & artery

Brachioradialis

Extensor carpi radialis longus

Pronator teres

Radius

Flexor digitorum profundus

Ulna

Extensor carpi ulnaris

Supinator

Extensor digitorum communis

Extensor carpi radialis brevis

Extensor pollicis longus

Extensor digiti minimi

Abductor pollicis longus

Extensor carpi radialis longus

Extensor carpi radialis brevis

Extensor digitorum communis

Extensor digiti minimi

Extensor carpi ulnaris

Supinator

Abductor pollicis longus

Extensor pollicis brevis

Extensor pollicis longus

Extensor indicis

ANTERIOR VIEW OF
SUPERFICIAL MUSCLES OF PALMAR HAND

ANTERIOR VIEW OF
DEEP MUSCLES OF PALMAR HAND

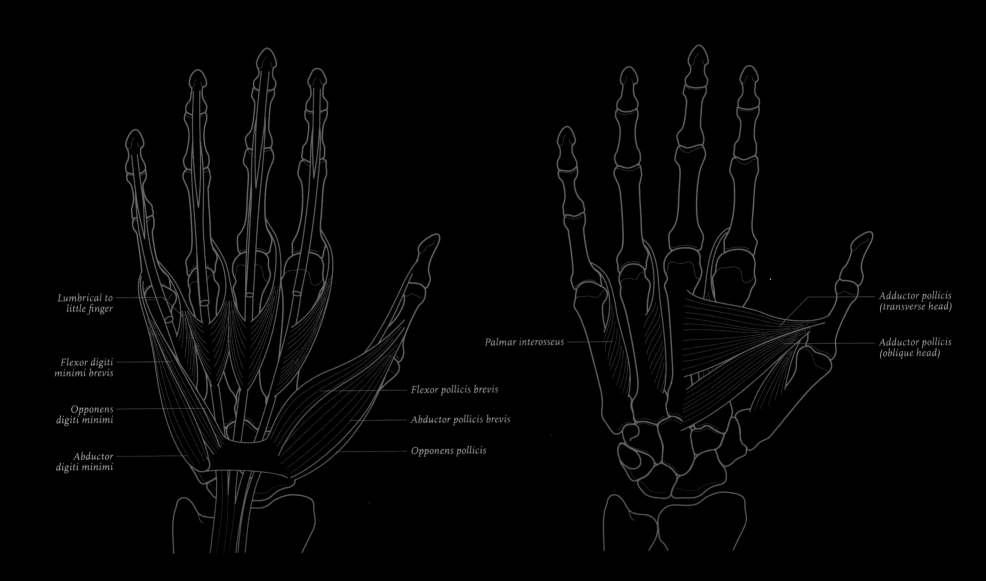

Lumbrical to
little finger

Flexor digiti
minimi brevis

Opponens
digiti minimi

Abductor
digiti minimi

Flexor pollicis brevis

Abductor pollicis brevis

Opponens pollicis

Adductor pollicis
(transverse head)

Palmar interosseus

Adductor pollicis
(oblique head)

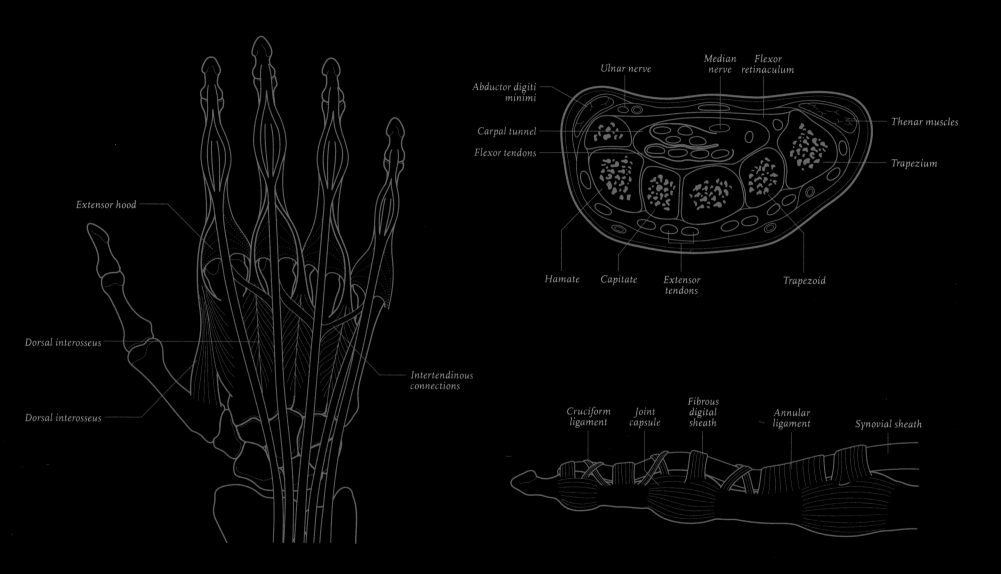

Ulnar nerve

Median
nerve

Flexor
retinaculum

Abductor digiti
minimi

Carpal tunnel

Flexor tendons

Thenar muscles

Trapezium

Extensor hood

Dorsal interosseus

Dorsal interosseus

Intertendinous
connections

Hamate

Capitate

Extensor
tendons

Trapezoid

Cruciform
ligament

Joint
capsule

Fibrous
digital
sheath

Annular
ligament

Synovial sheath

LATERAL VIEW OF DIGIT

Blood supply to the arm is via the brachial artery, a continuation of the axillary artery at the lower border of teres major muscle. Just below the elbow, it divides into ulnar and radial branches in the forearm, going on to form the deep and superficial palmar arches in the hands. Many collateral branches occur around joints to ensure that, if blood supply is occluded in one artery, blood can still reach tissues distal to the obstruction.

Venous drainage of the upper limb is by both superficial and deep veins. The superficial veins, although varying in pattern, are the basilic and cephalic veins. The deep veins, which tend to accompany the main arteries and travel in pairs known as the venae comitantes, communicate with the superficial veins.

The innervation of the muscles of the arm stems from the complex organisation of nerve roots, trunks and divisions of the brachial plexus. This arrangement terminates in five main nerves: the axillary, musculocutaneous, radial, median and ulnar nerves.

Additional branches are also given off, such as the long thoracic nerve (supplying serratus anterior), dorsal scapular nerve (rhomboids), suprascapular nerve (supraspinatus and infraspinatus), medial and lateral pectoral nerve (pectoralis major), thoracodorsal nerve (latissimus dorsi) and the upper and lower subscapular nerve (subscapularis and teres major).

The axillary nerve winds around the surgical neck of the humerus and supplies deltoid and teres minor and has a sensory function to the lateral part of the upper arm. The radial nerve lies on the posterior aspect of the humerus, travelling with the profunda brachii artery in the spiral groove, and supplies triceps brachii, brachioradialis and the extensor compartment of the forearm. It also receives sensory stimuli from the skin on the posterior aspect of the arm, forearm and dorsolateral hand.

The musculocutaneous nerve supplies coracobrachialis then passes between and supplies biceps brachii and brachialis. It then becomes cutaneous, as the lateral cutaneous nerve of the forearm, providing sensory innervation for the lateral forearm.

The median nerve travels with the brachial artery, eventually crossing it to lie medial to it before reaching the cubital fossa. It supplies all of the muscles in the anterior compartment of the forearm (except flexor carpi ulnaris and the ulnar half of flexor digitorum profundus), the thenar muscles and the two lateral lumbricals. Additionally, it is sensory to the skin over the lateral palm and three and a half digits.

Finally, the ulnar nerve supplies the remaining intrinsic muscles of the hand, flexor carpi ulnaris and the ulnar half of flexor digitorum profundus, and is sensory to the remaining palmar skin.

ANTERIOR VIEW OF
ARTERIES OF UPPER LIMB

ANTERIOR VIEW OF
VEINS OF UPPER LIMB

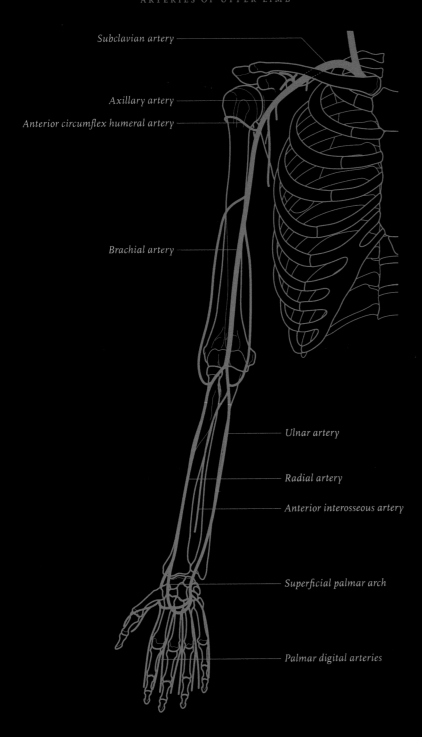

Subclavian artery

Axillary artery

Anterior circumflex humeral artery

Brachial artery

Ulnar artery

Radial artery

Anterior interosseous artery

Superficial palmar arch

Palmar digital arteries

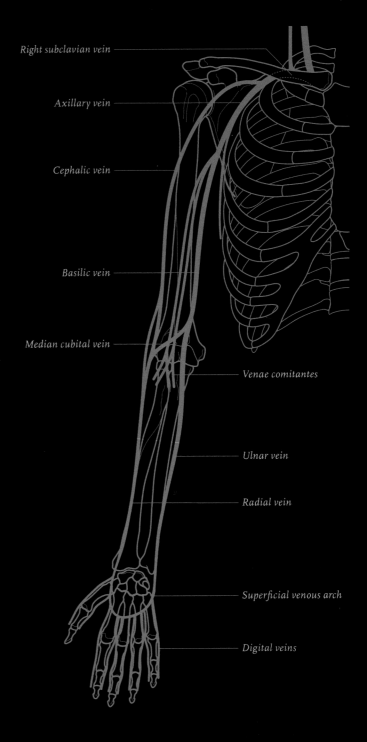

Right subclavian vein

Axillary vein

Cephalic vein

Basilic vein

Median cubital vein

Venae comitantes

Ulnar vein

Radial vein

Superficial venous arch

Digital veins

ANTERIOR VIEW OF CUBITAL FOSSA

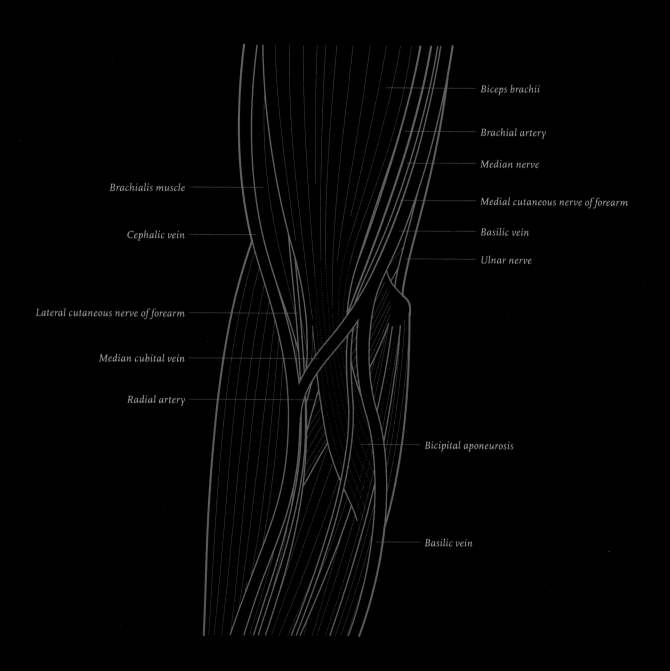

Biceps brachii

Brachial artery

Median nerve

Brachialis muscle

Medial cutaneous nerve of forearm

Cephalic vein

Basilic vein

Ulnar nerve

Lateral cutaneous nerve of forearm

Median cubital vein

Radial artery

Bicipital aponeurosis

Basilic vein

ANTERIOR VIEW OF BRACHIAL PLEXUS

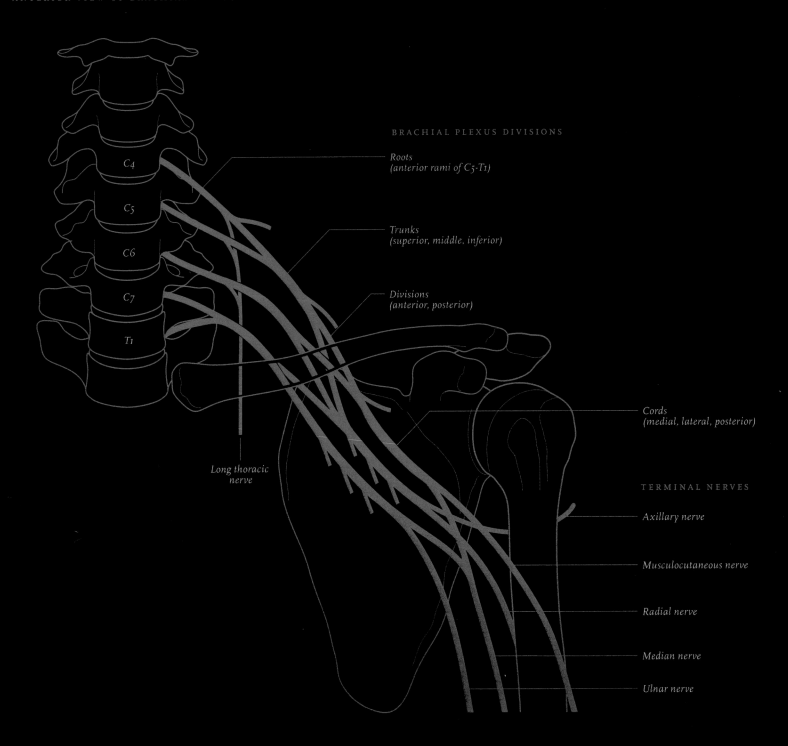

C4

C5

C6

C7

T1

BRACHIAL PLEXUS DIVISIONS

Roots
(anterior rami of C5-T1)

Trunks
(superior, middle, inferior)

Divisions
(anterior, posterior)

Cords
(medial, lateral, posterior)

Long thoracic
nerve

TERMINAL NERVES

Axillary nerve

Musculocutaneous nerve

Radial nerve

Median nerve

Ulnar nerve

ANTERIOR VIEW OF
NERVES OF UPPER LIMB

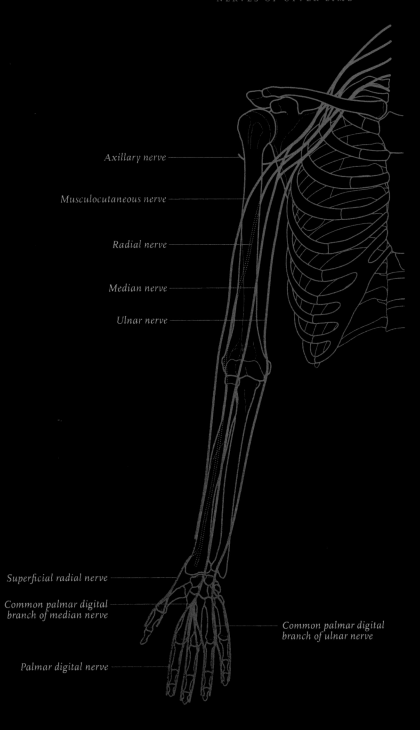

Axillary nerve

Musculocutaneous nerve

Radial nerve

Median nerve

Ulnar nerve

Superficial radial nerve

Common palmar digital
branch of median nerve

Common palmar digital
branch of ulnar nerve

Palmar digital nerve

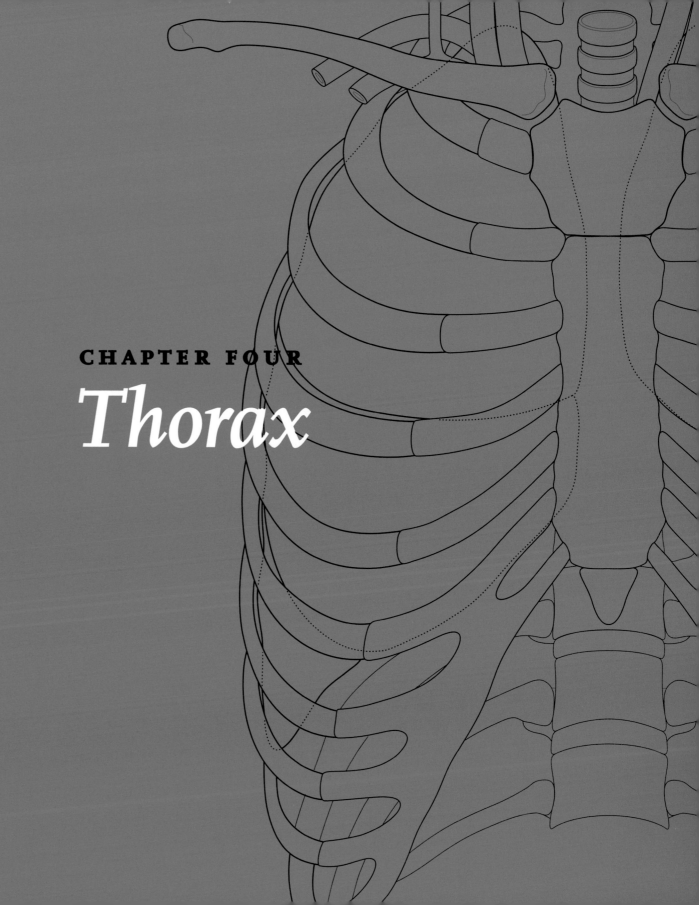

CHAPTER FOUR
Thorax

THE RIB CAGE & LUNGS

The bony thorax consists of twelve ribs on either side, each individually articulating with the thoracic vertebrae posteriorly and the sternum anteriorly via costal cartilages.

The sternum can be divided into the superior manubrium, which articulates with the body of the sternum via the fibrocartilaginous manubriosternal joint, and the xiphoid process, inferiorly articulating by the fibrocartilaginous xiphisternal joint. The costal cartilages of ribs 1–7 articulate directly with the sternum via their costal cartilages with synovial joints, hence they are called 'true ribs'. Ribs 8–10 articulate indirectly with the sternum via cartilages connecting to the seventh costal cartilage, hence they are termed 'false ribs'. The two 'floating ribs' 11 and 12 do not articulate with the sternum.

Posteriorly, ribs 2–9 form synovial joints with both the superior and transverse facets of their respective thoracic vertebrae and the inferior facet on the body of the vertebra above. Ribs 1 and 10–12 articulate only with their respective vertebrae, and ribs 11 and 12 have no costotransverse joints. Collective movements of the ribs upon the vertebral column assist in altering the volume of the thoracic cavity during breathing.

The space between the ribs is known as the intercostal space and contains three layers of muscles (external, internal and innermost intercostal muscles), plus vessels and nerves associated with each rib in the costal groove. Although the diaphragm provides the majority of the inspiratory effort, the remainder is provided via the external intercostals. The opposing direction of the fibres of the internal and innermost intercostals assists in expiration.

The thoracic inlet is formed by the first ribs, their costal cartilages, the manubrium of the sternum anteriorly and the first thoracic vertebra posteriorly. It transmits the oesophagus, trachea, nerves, ducts and vessels. The lung apices and pleurae project above the inlet and clavicles as the inlet slopes downwards anteriorly.

The right lung can be divided into three lobes (superior, middle, inferior) by the oblique and horizontal fissures. The left lung is smaller and has two lobes (superior and inferior) separated by the oblique fissure. It has a thin lingual ('tongue') part as it curves around the heart.

Both lungs are enveloped in pleura, a two-layered membrane. One layer is attached to the lung (visceral pleura), and the other parietal pleural layer lines the thoracic wall, diaphragmatic surface and pericardium. The two layers create a sealed pleural cavity containing serous fluid to decrease friction as the layers slide over one another. The two layers are continuous at the hilum of the lung, and leave a potential space between the diaphragm and the ribs for deep inspiration called the costodiaphragmatic recess.

The air supply to the lungs comes via the trachea, an elastic tube held open by 'C'-shaped rings of cartilage. At the hila of the lungs, the trachea divides into a left and right bronchus, the left being more horizontal than the right. The bronchi further divide into collective groups supplying a specific segment of the lung (bronchopulmonary segment). Segmental bronchi branch into several bronchioles, which lead to respiratory bronchioles and end in a blind alveolar sac where gas exchange takes place through a capillary network covering the alveoli, exchanging carbon dioxide in the blood for oxygen.

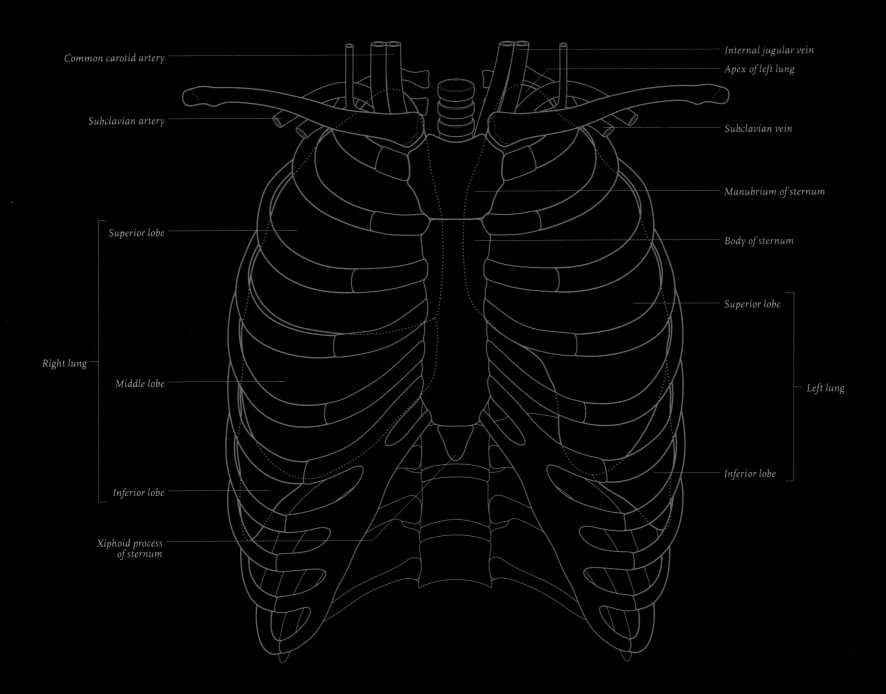

Common carotid artery

Subclavian artery

Superior lobe

Right lung

Middle lobe

Inferior lobe

Xiphoid process
of sternum

Internal jugular vein

Apex of left lung

Subclavian vein

Manubrium of sternum

Body of sternum

Superior lobe

Left lung

Inferior lobe

ANTERIOR VIEW OF RIBCAGE

POSTERIOR VIEW OF RIBCAGE

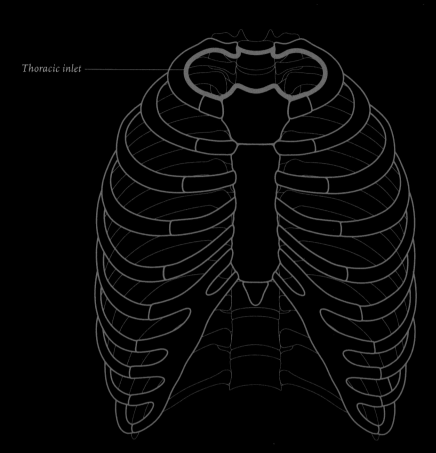

Thoracic inlet

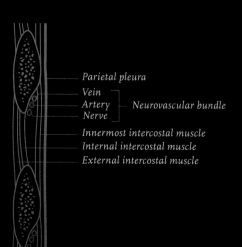

Parietal pleura

Vein
Artery   *Neurovascular bundle*
Nerve

Innermost intercostal muscle
Internal intercostal muscle
External intercostal muscle

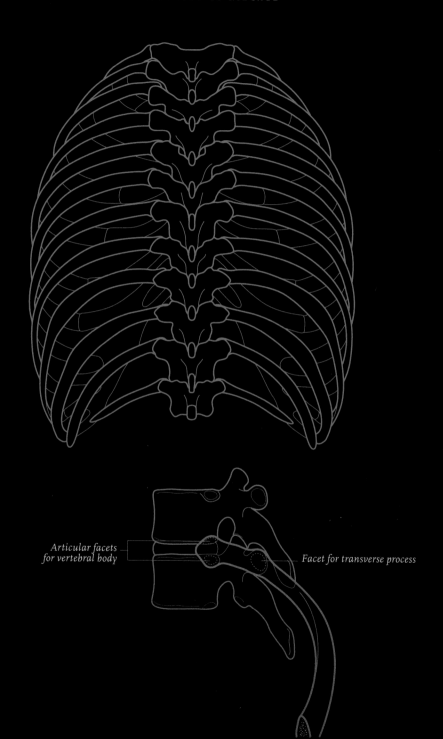

Articular facets for vertebral body

Facet for transverse process

ANTERIOR VIEW OF LUNGS AND TRACHEA

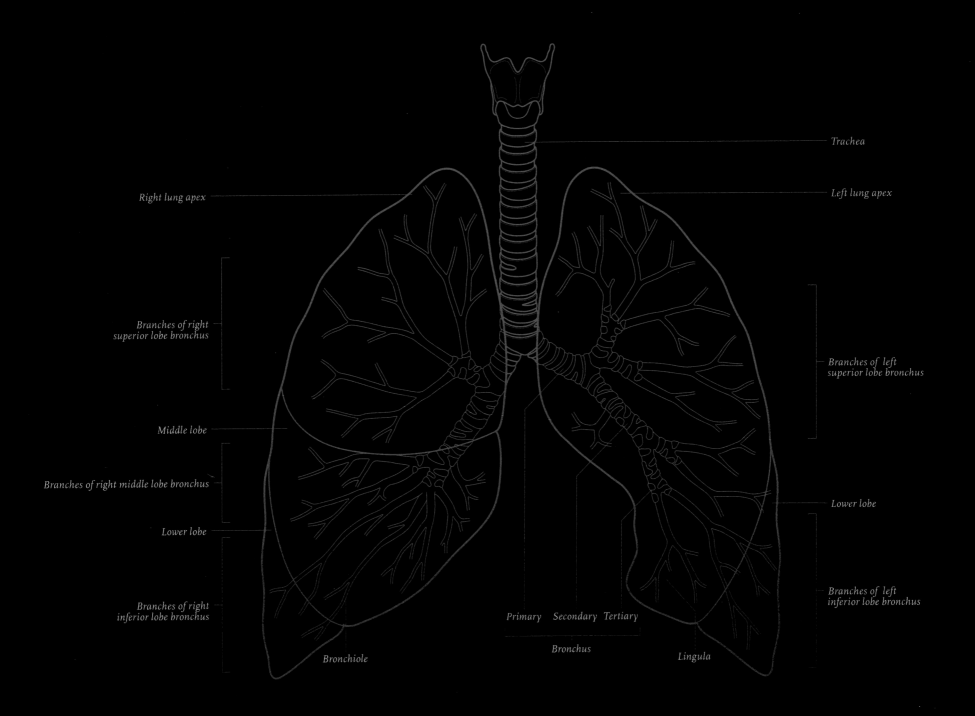

Trachea

Right lung apex

Left lung apex

Branches of right
superior lobe bronchus

Branches of left
superior lobe bronchus

Middle lobe

Branches of right middle lobe bronchus

Lower lobe

Lower lobe

Branches of right
inferior lobe bronchus

Branches of left
inferior lobe bronchus

Primary   Secondary   Tertiary

Bronchus

Bronchiole

Lingula

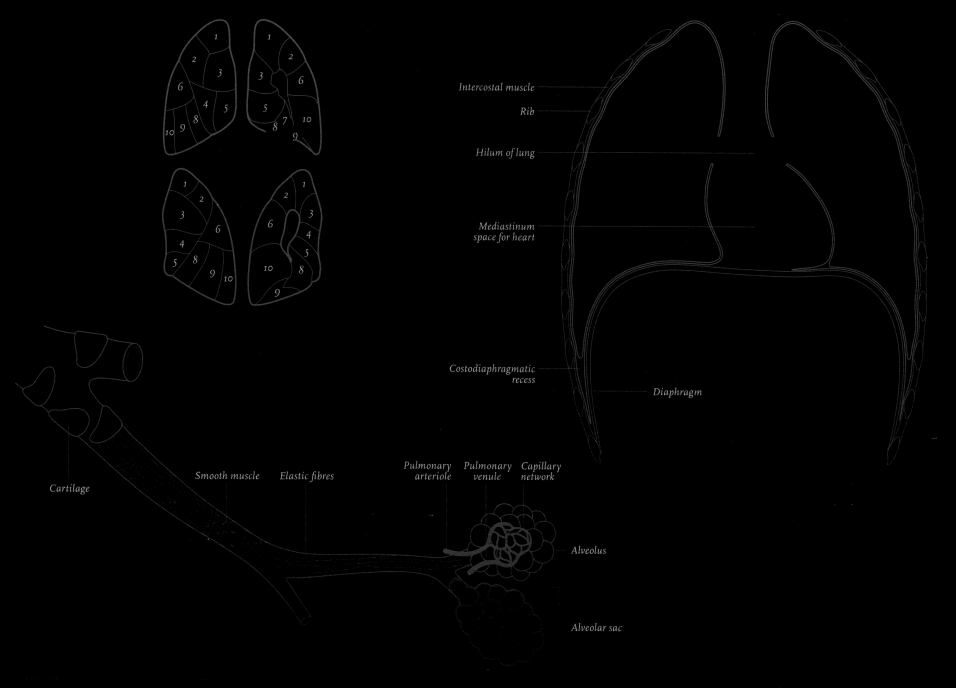

Intercostal muscle

Rib

Hilum of lung

Mediastinum
space for heart

Costodiaphragmatic
recess

Diaphragm

Cartilage

Smooth muscle

Elastic fibres

Pulmonary
arteriole

Pulmonary
venule

Capillary
network

Alveolus

Alveolar sac

Bronchi

Bronchiole

THE MEDIASTINUM & HEART

The mediastinum is the area in the centre of the thoracic cavity between the lungs. It can be divided into superior and inferior regions.

The superior mediastinum has a superior boundary of the thoracic inlet, and an inferior boundary of a transverse plane that passes between the manubriosternal joint to the T4/5 intervertebral disc. The inferior mediastinum lies beneath this plane and continues as far as the diaphragm. It can be divided into anterior (between the sternum and heart), middle (heart) and posterior (between heart and thoracic vertebrae) compartments.

The heart lies in a three-layered sac called the pericardium. The outer fibrous pericardial layer is fused to the great vessels, sternum and diaphragm. Beneath this layer lies the parietal layer that reflects onto the heart and becomes the visceral layer. Between the two is the pericardial cavity containing serous fluid. The mechanics of this structure allows the heart to beat smoothly, prevents overfilling and reduces movement within the middle mediastinum. It receives sensory fibres from the phrenic nerve.

The walls of the heart consist of cardiac muscle lined with endothelium formed into four chambers. It can be divided into the pulmonary heart on the right side, whose two chambers collect deoxygenated blood from the body and pump it to the lungs to be oxygenated, and the systemic heart on the left side, which takes the oxygenated blood from the lungs and pumps it to the rest of the body.

The thin-walled right atrium collects blood from the superior vena cava (draining the upper body), inferior vena cava (draining the lower body) and coronary sinus (draining venous blood from the heart walls). Its smooth medial wall is home to a feature called the fossa ovalis, which is a remnant of fetal circulation when blood flow would bypass the lungs and go directly from right atrium to left. Atrial contraction causes the blood to pass into the right ventricle through the tricuspid valve. This chamber has thick irregular muscular walls with ridges called trabeculae carneae. Some of these are larger than others (papillary muscles) and attach at their superior end to fibres (chordae tendineae) that prevent them blowing back into the atria by adhering to the tricuspid valve cusps. The blood is then forced up through the smooth-walled conus arteriosus, through the semilunar pulmonary valve into the pulmonary trunk and subsequently pulmonary arteries to the lungs. The left atrium then receives the oxygenated blood from the lungs via the pulmonary veins and, during atrial contraction, passes it to the left ventricle through the bicuspid (mitral) valve. The left ventricular wall is thicker than the right as it pumps blood at a higher pressure than its counterpart. Blood

passes through the semilunar aortic valve to the aortic arch to take blood to the body. Just above the aortic valve are the coronary sinuses that give off the left and right coronary arteries, which in turn branch into a series of small arteries supplying the heart muscle with arterial blood.

Coordination of the contraction of the heart is achieved by electrical impulses from the conduction system. A collection of specialised cells, called the sinuatrial node, in the wall of the right atrium initiates the contraction of the atrium, and is therefore called the 'pacemaker'. The electrical impulses spread across both atria and cause them to contract. The atrioventricular node detects this impulse and directs it to a system of conduction tissue called the atrioventricular bundle, which is continuous with the Purkinje fibres. These spread the electrical impulse to the muscular tissue in the ventricular muscle tissue causing it to contract. The sounds of the blood flow through the heart can be detected through auscultation (listening with a stethoscope) at various sites on the chest wall.

Although contraction of cardiac muscle occurs without motor nerves, the vagus nerve can decrease cardiac output through parasympathetic innervation, and branches from the sympathetic chain to the cardiac plexus increase cardiac output.

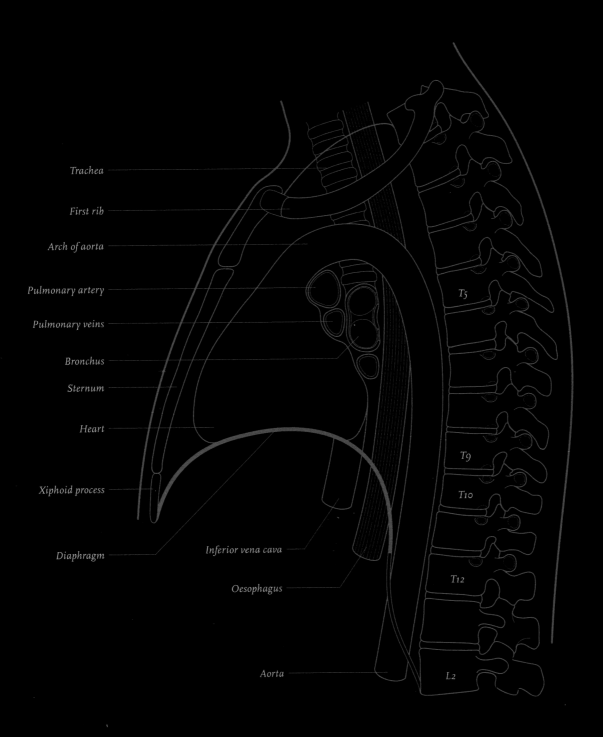

Trachea

First rib

Arch of aorta

Pulmonary artery

Pulmonary veins

Bronchus

Sternum

Heart

Xiphoid process

Diaphragm

Inferior vena cava

Oesophagus

Aorta

T5

T9

T10

T12

L2

TRANSVERSE SECTION THROUGH MEDIASTINUM

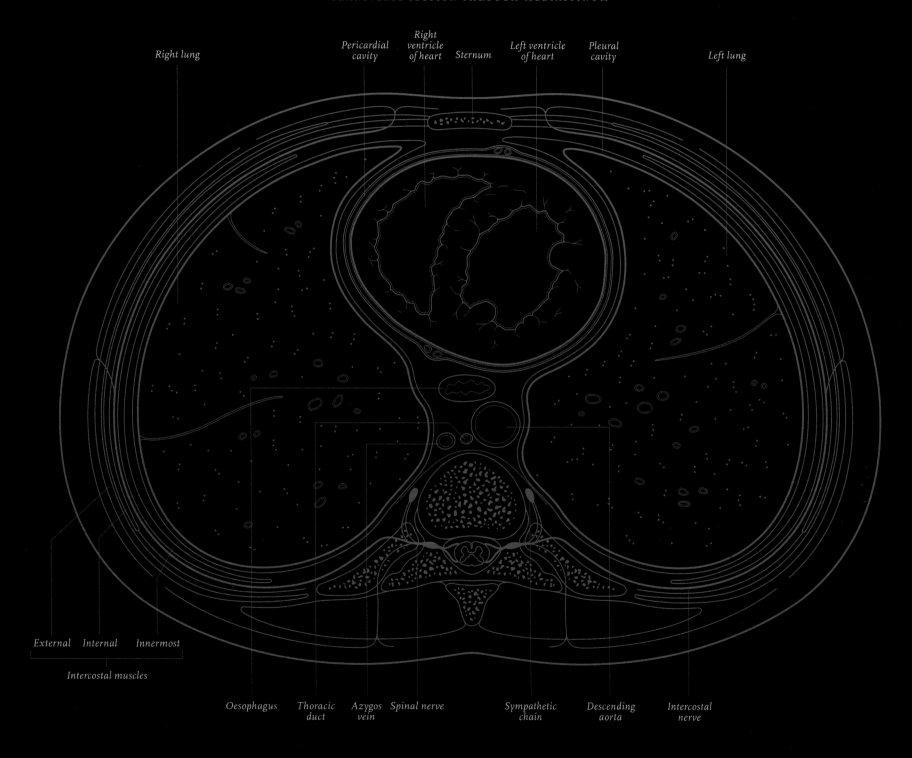

Right lung

Pericardial cavity

Right ventricle of heart

Sternum

Left ventricle of heart

Pleural cavity

Left lung

External   Internal   Innermost

Intercostal muscles

Oesophagus

Thoracic duct

Azygos vein

Spinal nerve

Sympathetic chain

Descending aorta

Intercostal nerve

ANTERIOR VIEW OF HEART

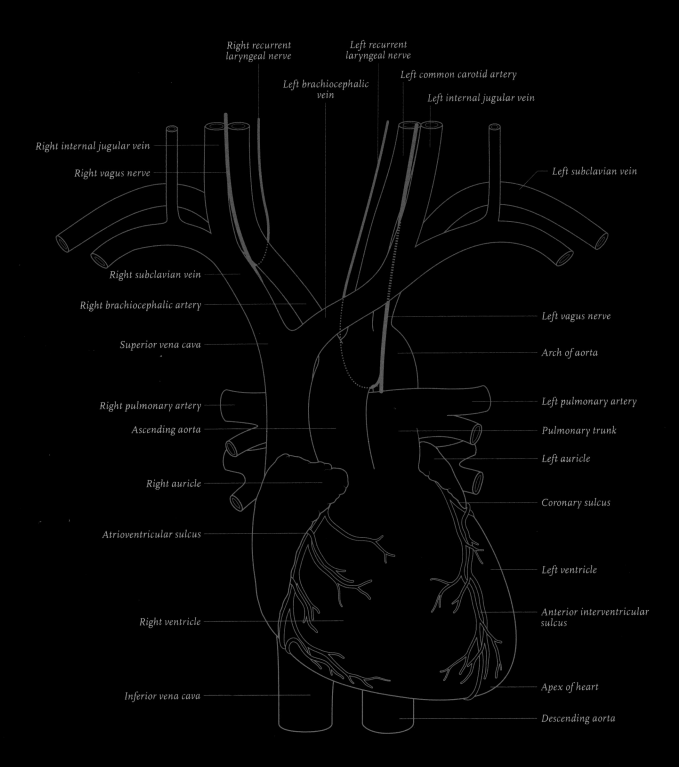

Right recurrent
laryngeal nerve

Left recurrent
laryngeal nerve

Left brachiocephalic
vein

Left common carotid artery

Left internal jugular vein

Right internal jugular vein

Right vagus nerve

Left subclavian vein

Right subclavian vein

Right brachiocephalic artery

Left vagus nerve

Superior vena cava

Arch of aorta

Right pulmonary artery

Left pulmonary artery

Ascending aorta

Pulmonary trunk

Left auricle

Right auricle

Coronary sulcus

Atrioventricular sulcus

Left ventricle

Right ventricle

Anterior interventricular
sulcus

Inferior vena cava

Apex of heart

Descending aorta

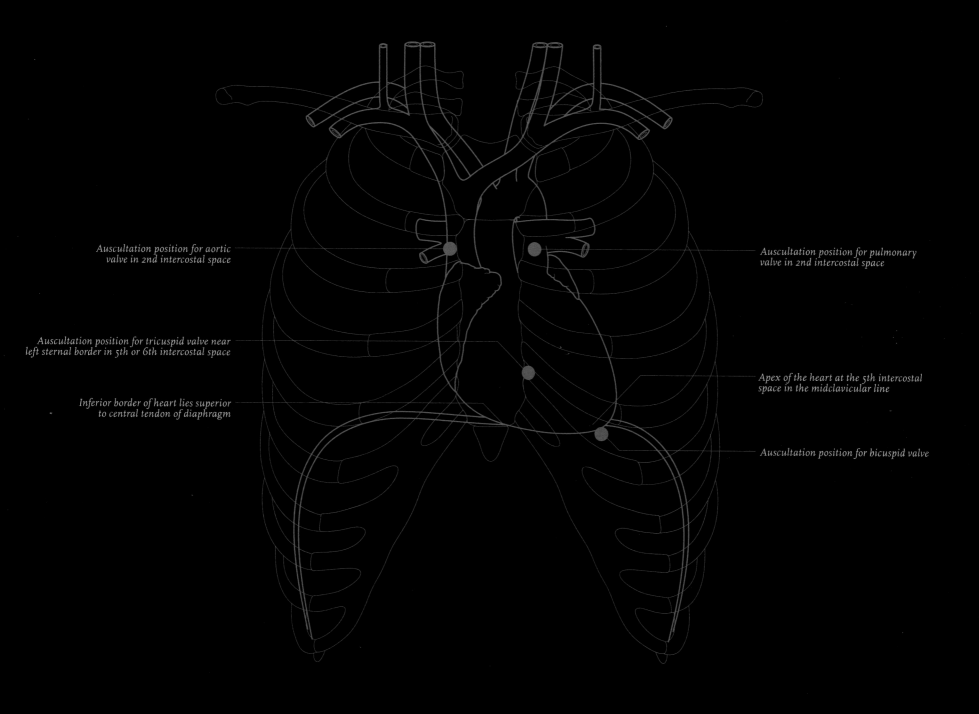

Auscultation position for aortic
valve in 2nd intercostal space

Auscultation position for pulmonary
valve in 2nd intercostal space

Auscultation position for tricuspid valve near
left sternal border in 5th or 6th intercostal space

Apex of the heart at the 5th intercostal
space in the midclavicular line

Inferior border of heart lies superior
to central tendon of diaphragm

Auscultation position for bicuspid valve

ANTERIOR VIEW OF CHAMBERS OF HEART

TRANSVERSE SECTION THROUGH VENTRICLES

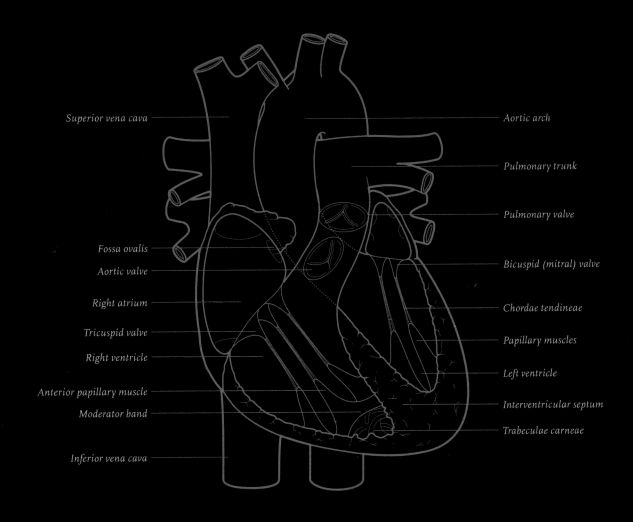

Superior vena cava

Fossa ovalis

Aortic valve

Right atrium

Tricuspid valve

Right ventricle

Anterior papillary muscle

Moderator band

Inferior vena cava

Aortic arch

Pulmonary trunk

Pulmonary valve

Bicuspid (mitral) valve

Chordae tendineae

Papillary muscles

Left ventricle

Interventricular septum

Trabeculae carneae

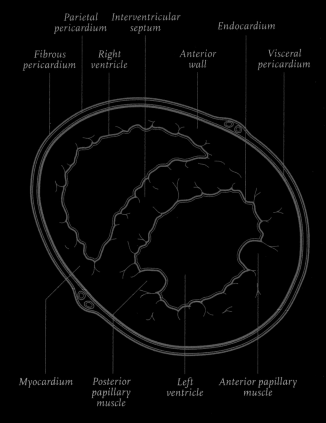

Parietal
pericardium

Interventricular
septum

Endocardium

Fibrous
pericardium

Right
ventricle

Anterior
wall

Visceral
pericardium

Myocardium

Posterior
papillary
muscle

Left
ventricle

Anterior papillary
muscle

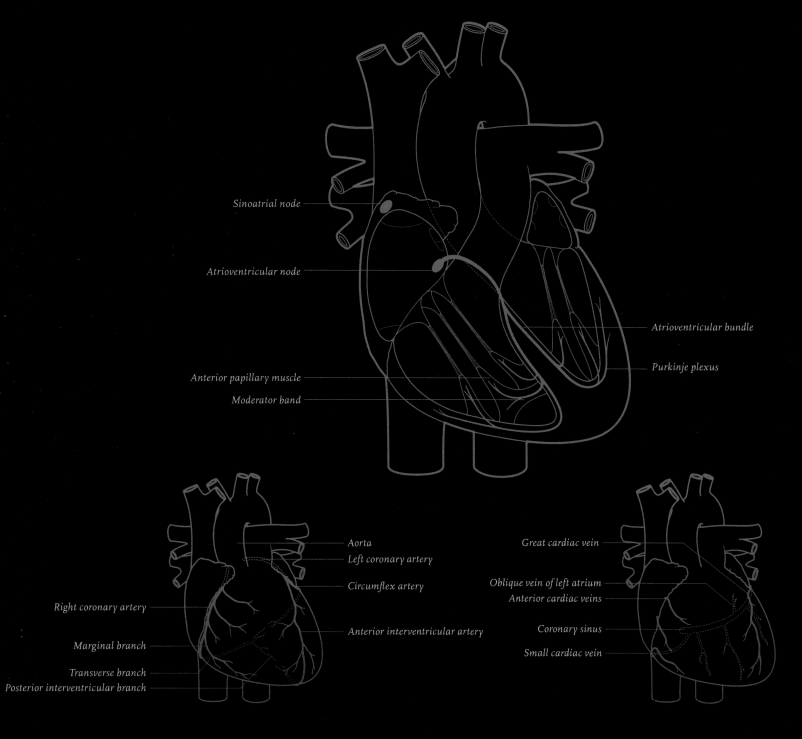

Sinoatrial node

Atrioventricular node

Atrioventricular bundle

Purkinje plexus

Anterior papillary muscle

Moderator band

Aorta
Left coronary artery

Circumflex artery

Right coronary artery

Anterior interventricular artery

Marginal branch

Transverse branch
Posterior interventricular branch

Great cardiac vein

Oblique vein of left atrium
Anterior cardiac veins

Coronary sinus

Small cardiac vein

CARDIAC ARTERIAL SUPPLY

CARDIAC VENOUS DRAINAGE

THE THORACIC WALL

The intercostal spaces are supplied by the anterior and posterior intercostal arteries. The posterior intercostal arteries for rib spaces 3–11 come directly from the thoracic aorta (those for ribs 1 and 2 come from the costocervical trunk). The anterior intercostals originate from the internal thoracic arteries (branches of the subclavian artery) and connect with the posterior arteries. Intercostal veins follow a similar rule, although the posterior intercostals drain into the azygos system. Nervous supply to the thoracic wall is by way of spinal nerves and contributions from the sympathetic chain, which runs either side of the vertebral column and supplies the intercostal muscle and skin of the same vertebral level (T1–T12).

Lymphatic capillaries collect excess fluid from around cells and tissues and merge, forming progressively larger lymph vessels that drain into veins in the neck. Lying on the anterior surface of the thoracic vertebrae is the thoracic duct, which is a continuation of the cisterna chyli (a dilated lymph sac that collects lymph from the intestinal and lumbar lymph trunks). It ascends to drain into the left subclavian vein at its junction with the internal jugular vein. On the right side, the right lymph duct drains the right side of the body as far as the abdomen. Lymph filtering units called lymph nodes can be found at the site of certain lymph vessels. Superficial nodes can be freely palpated, such as some axillary nodes. The presence of lymphatic vessels in the breast is

significant as they drain the fat portion of the milk produced in lactation; additionally they transfer infected material away from the breast.

During puberty, the increase in oestrogen causes breast tissue to enlarge. This is mostly composed of fatty tissue with associated vessels and suspensory ligaments overlying the pectoralis muscle on the anterior thoracic wall. Pregnancy triggers the development of the lactiferous duct system and associated glandular tissue. In the latter stages of pregnancy, the glands start producing milk, which is collected by ducts that converge at lactiferous sinuses before it is excreted from the nipple.

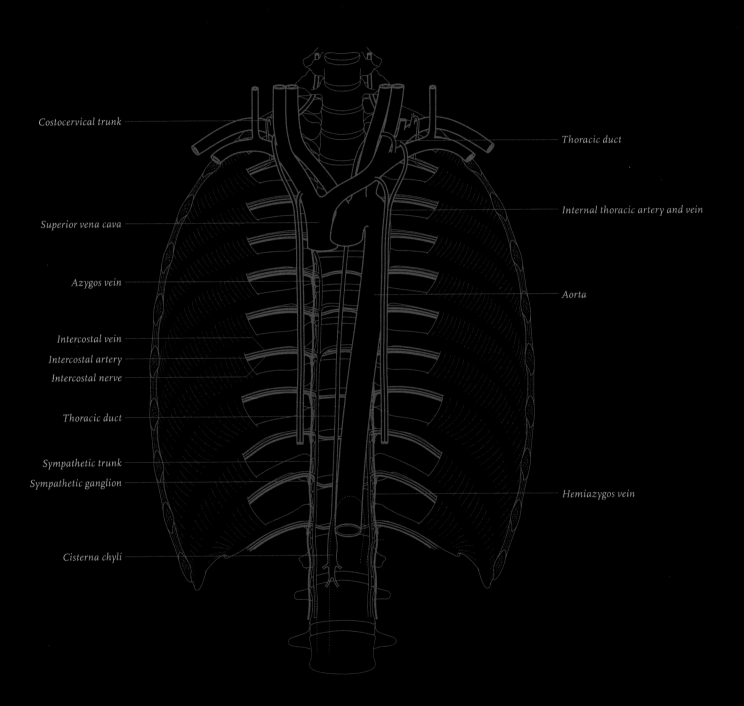

Costocervical trunk

Superior vena cava

Azygos vein

Intercostal vein

Intercostal artery

Intercostal nerve

Thoracic duct

Sympathetic trunk

Sympathetic ganglion

Cisterna chyli

Thoracic duct

Internal thoracic artery and vein

Aorta

Hemiazygos vein

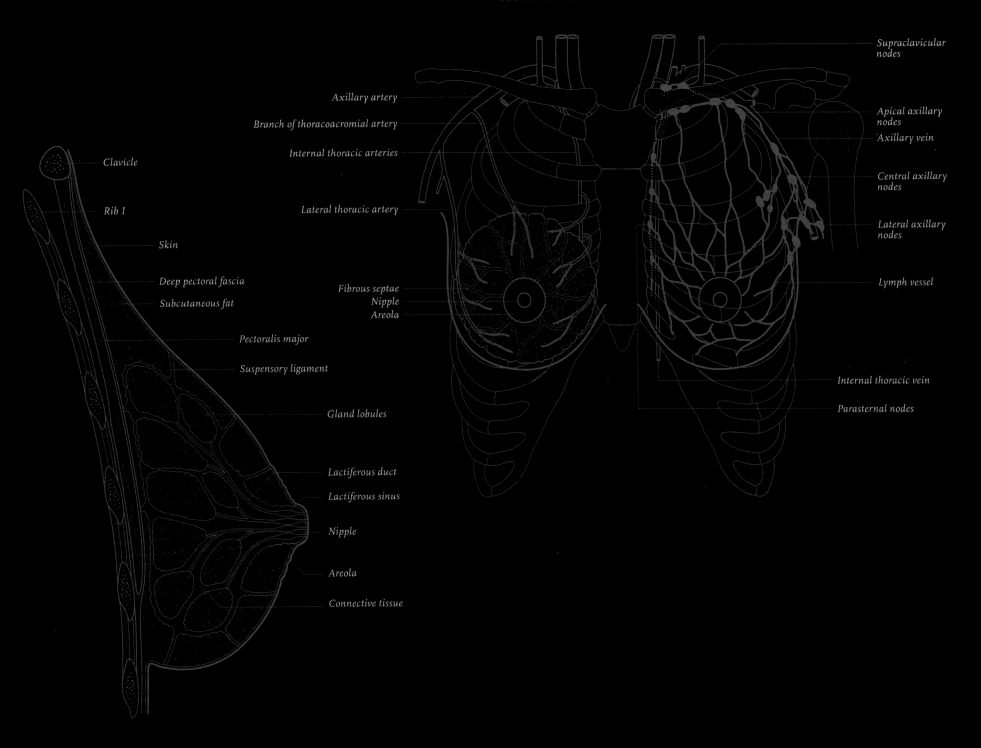

Supraclavicular nodes

Axillary artery

Branch of thoracoacromial artery

Internal thoracic arteries

Apical axillary nodes

Axillary vein

Lateral thoracic artery

Central axillary nodes

Lateral axillary nodes

Fibrous septae
Nipple
Areola

Lymph vessel

Clavicle

Rib I

Skin

Deep pectoral fascia

Subcutaneous fat

Pectoralis major

Suspensory ligament

Gland lobules

Internal thoracic vein

Parasternal nodes

Lactiferous duct

Lactiferous sinus

Nipple

Areola

Connective tissue

SAGITTAL SECTION THROUGH BREAST

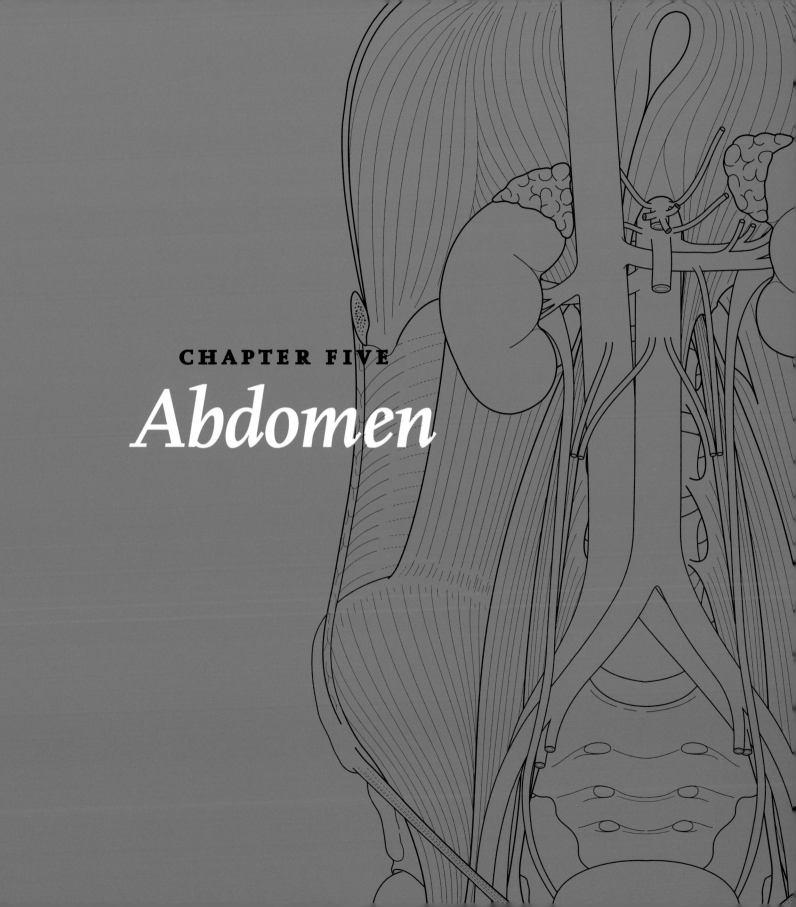

CHAPTER FIVE
Abdomen

THE ABDOMINAL WALL & CAVITY

The abdomen is the area between the diaphragm superiorly and the pelvis inferiorly. It has muscular anterior and posterior abdominal walls, which are anchored to the lumbar vertebrae, ribs and pelvis. Anteriorly, the three thin muscle layers of transversus abdominis, and internal and external oblique retain the viscera within the abdominal cavity and act to compress the abdominal contents during expiration, urination and defaecation. The tendons (aponeuroses) of all three invest the main flexor of the trunk, rectus abdominis, anteriorly and merge at the midline to form the linea alba.

The inguinal canal is a region just above the inguinal ligament on the anteroinferior abdominal wall. It carries the spermatic cord in males and the round ligament in females. During development, as the testes migrate from the abdominal cavity to the scrotum, they push through the layers of the anterior abdominal wall, of which each layer then constitutes a layer of the spermatic cord. The remaining deep and superficial rings are potential areas of weakness in the abdominal wall as a result.

The diaphragm separates the viscera of the thorax from those of the abdomen. It originates from the lumbar vertebral bodies as the left (L1–L2) and right (L1–L3) crura, and the arcuate ligaments, as well as the lower six ribs and the xiphisternum. The muscle fibres converge as one central tendon, which is fused with the fibrous pericardium and is supplied by the phrenic nerve. The aorta, oesophagus, inferior vena cava, lymph vessels and vagal/sympathetic nerve fibres pass through apertures in the diaphragm to the abdomen.

Posteriorly, quadratus lumborum (an extensor of the lumbar vertebrae) and two psoas major muscles (powerful flexors of the lumbar spine and hip joint) form the muscles of the posterior abdominal wall.

The abdominal cavity is lined with a serous membrane called parietal peritoneum, which is reflected off the abdominal wall onto the viscera as visceral peritoneum. As the intestines invaginate into the cavity, the double-sided folds of peritoneum enclosing their vessels and nerve supply are called mesenteries. The viscera that are suspended on a mesentery are the stomach, jejunum, ileum, and transverse and sigmoid colon. The remaining structures are covered in peritoneum but are adherent to the posterior abdominal wall, and so are termed retroperitoneal. These include the aorta, inferior vena cava, kidneys, pancreas, duodenum, and ascending and descending colon. A large fatty fold of peritoneum, called the greater omentum, hangs from the stomach and transverse colon and usually covers the visible contents of the abdomen beneath the anterior abdominal wall. The potential space around the viscera in the peritoneal cavity is referred to as the greater sac, with the exception of space formed behind the stomach owing to the lesser omentum between the liver and stomach, which is called the lesser sac.

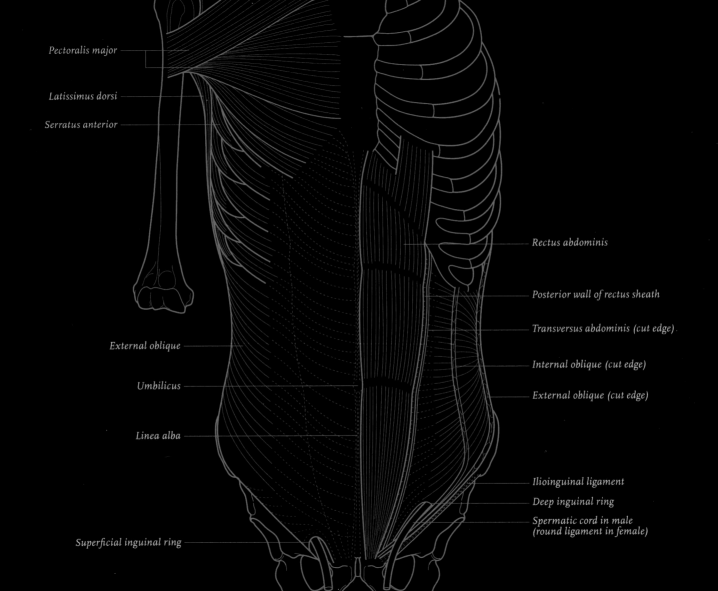

Pectoralis major

Latissimus dorsi

Serratus anterior

External oblique

Umbilicus

Linea alba

Superficial inguinal ring

Rectus abdominis

Posterior wall of rectus sheath

Transversus abdominis (cut edge)

Internal oblique (cut edge)

External oblique (cut edge)

Ilioinguinal ligament

Deep inguinal ring

Spermatic cord in male
(round ligament in female)

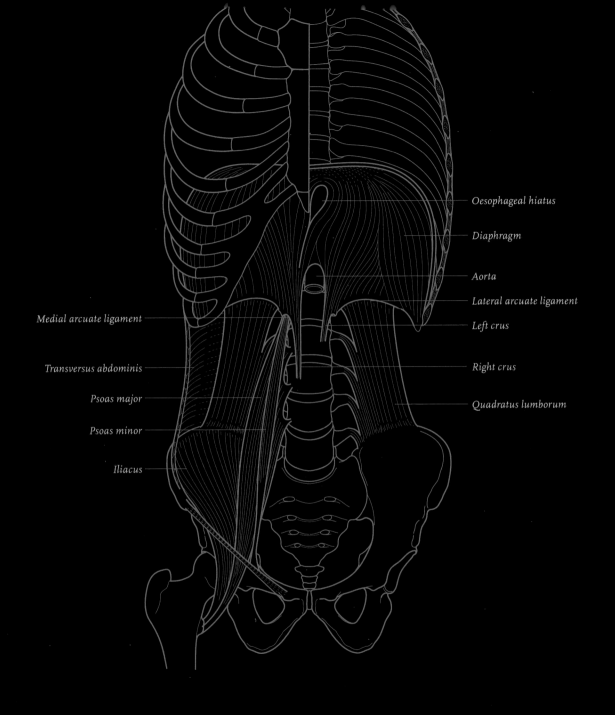

Oesophageal hiatus

Diaphragm

Aorta

Lateral arcuate ligament

Medial arcuate ligament

Left crus

Transversus abdominis

Right crus

Psoas major

Quadratus lumborum

Psoas minor

Iliacus

ANTERIOR VIEW OF PERITONEAL CAVITY

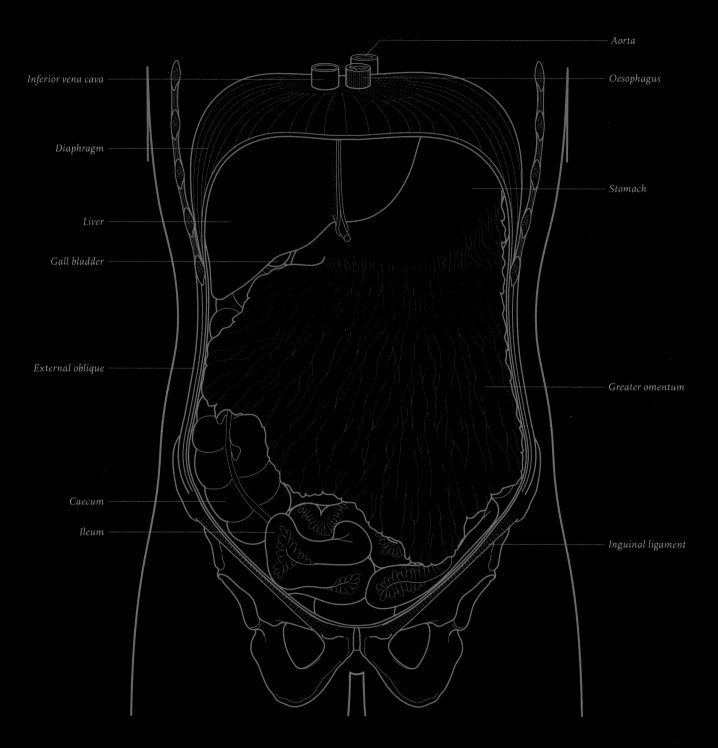

Inferior vena cava

Diaphragm

Liver

Gall bladder

External oblique

Caecum

Ileum

Aorta

Oesophagus

Stomach

Greater omentum

Inguinal ligament

ANTERIOR VIEW OF ABDOMINAL VISCERA

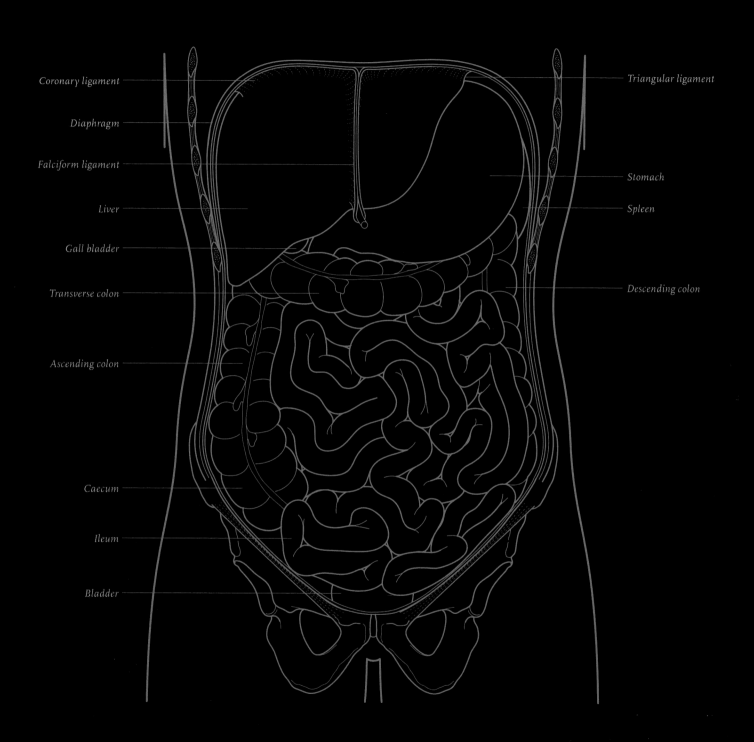

Coronary ligament

Diaphragm

Falciform ligament

Liver

Gall bladder

Transverse colon

Ascending colon

Caecum

Ileum

Bladder

Triangular ligament

Stomach

Spleen

Descending colon

TRANSVERSE VIEW THROUGH TRANSPYLORIC PLANE

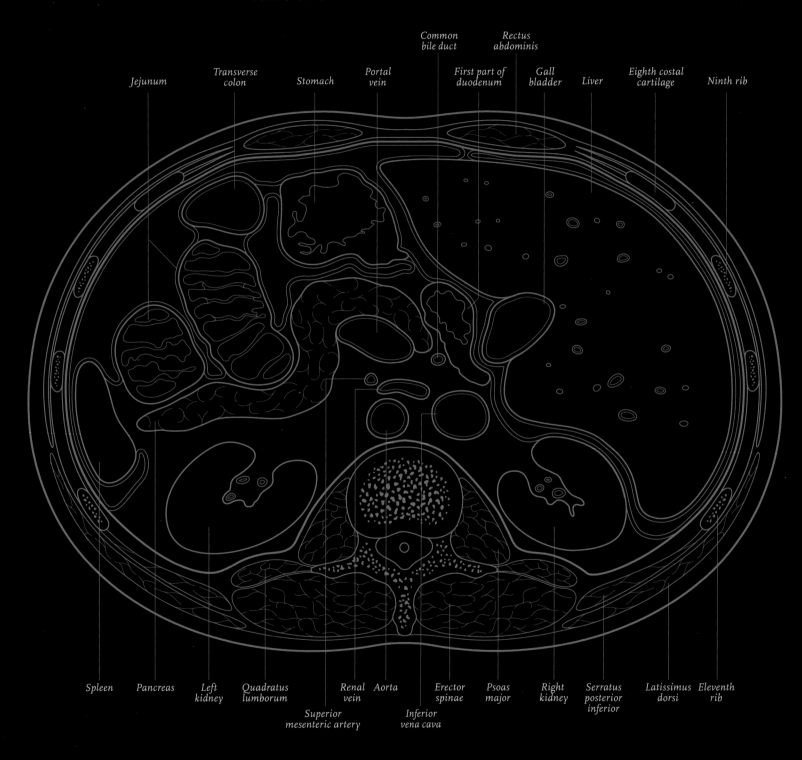

SAGITTAL SECTION THROUGH ABDOMINAL CAVITY

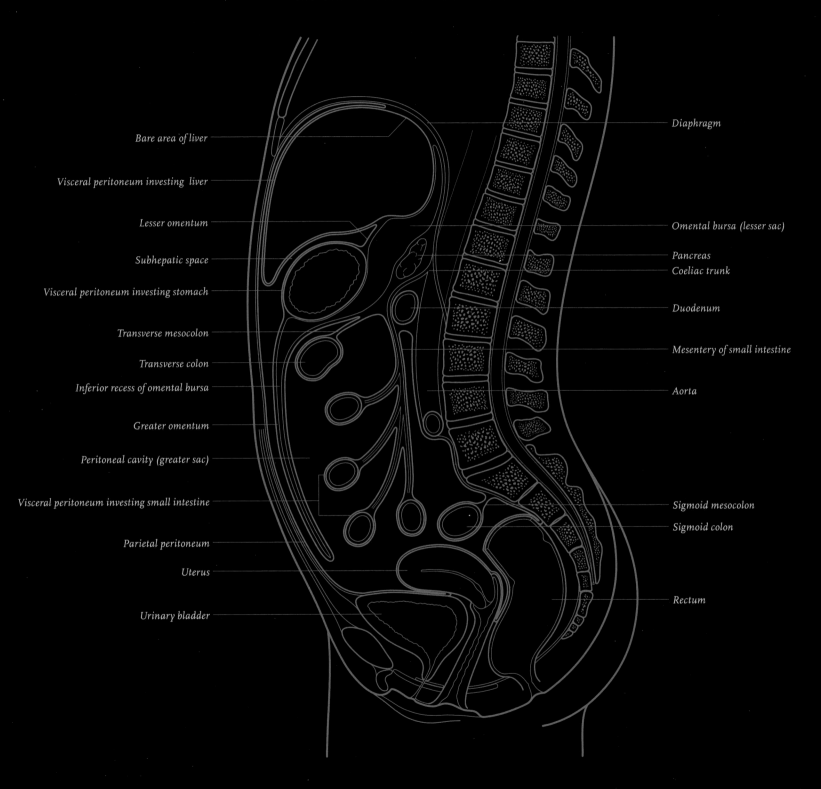

Bare area of liver

Visceral peritoneum investing liver

Lesser omentum

Subhepatic space

Visceral peritoneum investing stomach

Transverse mesocolon

Transverse colon

Inferior recess of omental bursa

Greater omentum

Peritoneal cavity (greater sac)

Visceral peritoneum investing small intestine

Parietal peritoneum

Uterus

Urinary bladder

Diaphragm

Omental bursa (lesser sac)

Pancreas
Coeliac trunk

Duodenum

Mesentery of small intestine

Aorta

Sigmoid mesocolon
Sigmoid colon

Rectum

THE STOMACH, INTESTINES & LIVER

The oesophagus passes through the diaphragm into the abdomen and joins with the stomach at the gastro-oesophageal junction. Here, at the area known as the cardia, a physiological sphincter relaxes during swallowing. The stomach is a dilated part of the gut whose muscular wall serves to mix food by peristalsis with digestive juices. Its mucosal surface is formed of a series of irregular folds called rugae. Partly digested food makes its way to the pyloric canal of the stomach before passing through the pyloric sphincter into the duodenum.

The duodenum is a retroperitoneal 'C'-shaped tube, which curves around the head of the pancreas receiving digestive juices from the pancreas and bile from the gall bladder via the duodenal papilla. It ascends superiorly to continue as the jejunum at the duodenojejunal junction, whilst becoming suspended by the common mesentery. Gradual changes in intestinal characteristics occur, as the jejunum becomes the ileum, throughout the convoluted route of the muscular tube. Mucosal folds called plicae circulares that increase the surface area for chemical digestion start to become less frequent in the ileum. The intestinal wall becomes thinner, pinker and narrower, and is supplied by blood vessels with more arcades and shorter straight arteries (vasa recta).

The large intestine extends from the caecum to the anus and has a primary role in reabsorbing

the water and electrolytes from the liquid that enters the caecum at the ileocaecal junction. Various defining features of the large intestine make it easily distinguishable from the small intestine. It has a band of longitudinal muscle called taenia coli that is shorter than the length of the wall, thus forces large sacculations (haustra) that are visible bulges in the intestinal wall. Another distinctive feature is the presence of small tags of fat attached to the intestinal wall, called appendices epiploicae, on the ascending, transverse and descending portions. As the sigmoid colon turns inferiorly to become the rectum, it loses these three features. The appendix originates at the caecum at the base of the taenia coli band, and is suspended from the terminal ileum by its own mesentery, the mesoappendix.

Arterial supply comes directly from the abdominal aorta as three main branches. The viscera supplied by the branches can be traced back to development of the gut. The foregut (stomach, part of duodenum, pancreas, spleen, liver, gall bladder) is supplied by branches of the coeliac trunk. The midgut (distal part of duodenum, jejunum, ileum, ascending and two-thirds of the transverse colon) is supplied by branches of the superior mesenteric artery. The hindgut (distal third of transverse colon, descending and sigmoid colon, rectum) is supplied by branches of the inferior mesenteric artery.

The venous drainage of the stomach, intestines and associated viscera is via the portal venous system. This takes the nutrient-rich blood from the digestive tract and delivers it to the liver for processing.

The liver is the largest visceral organ in the body. It is enveloped in visceral peritoneum, which reflects onto the inferior surface of the diaphragm around the bare area of the liver that is in contact with the diaphragm. These reflections are called coronary ligaments, and their edges termed triangular ligaments. Anteriorly, two layers of coronary ligament join to form the falciform ligament, which is continuous with the parietal peritoneum of the anterior abdominal wall. The liver comprises four lobes: the left, right, caudate and quadrate lobes. It receives arterial blood from the hepatic artery, a branch of the coeliac trunk. This artery, together with the portal vein, enters the liver at the porta hepatis. The other structure at the porta hepatis is the bile duct, which transmits bile either from its storage in the gall bladder (if large quantities are needed), or directly from hepatic ducts after its manufacture by hepatocytes in the liver.

Arterial, venous and biliary vessels are arranged segmentally in the liver. Venous drainage of the liver occurs segmentally through the hepatic veins into the inferior vena cava.

SAGITTAL SECTION THROUGH STOMACH

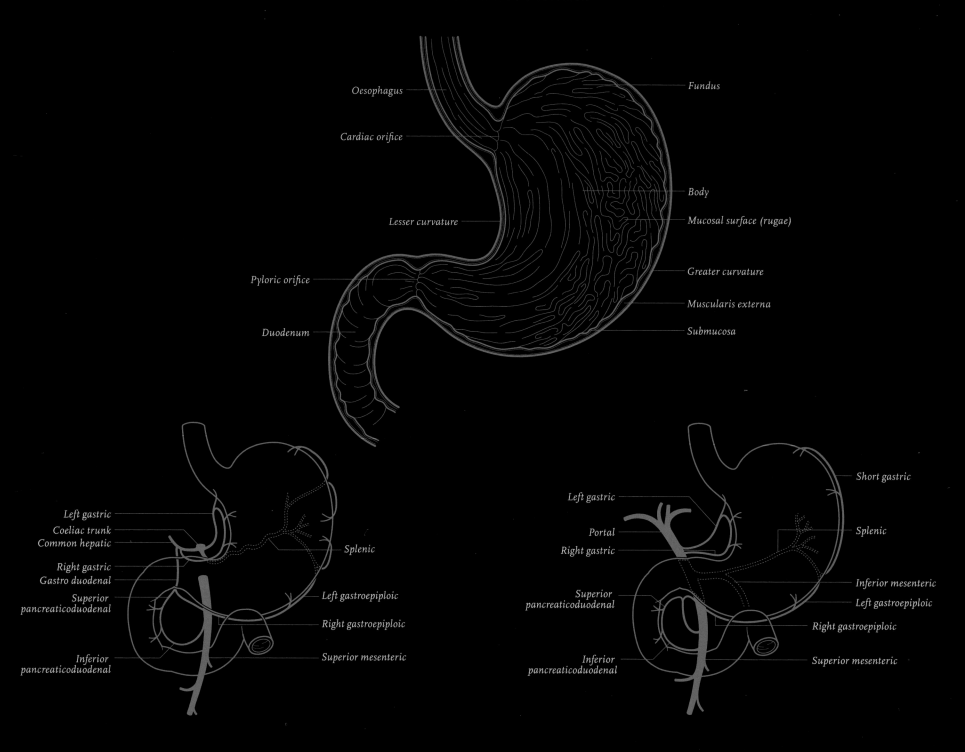

Oesophagus

Fundus

Cardiac orifice

Body

Lesser curvature

Mucosal surface (rugae)

Pyloric orifice

Greater curvature

Muscularis externa

Duodenum

Submucosa

Left gastric

Short gastric

Coeliac trunk

Left gastric

Common hepatic

Portal

Splenic

Right gastric

Right gastric

Splenic

Gastro duodenal

Superior
pancreaticoduodenal

Inferior mesenteric

Superior
pancreaticoduodenal

Left gastroepiploic

Left gastroepiploic

Right gastroepiploic

Right gastroepiploic

Inferior
pancreaticoduodenal

Superior mesenteric

Inferior
pancreaticoduodenal

Superior mesenteric

ARTERIAL SUPPLY OF STOMACH

VENOUS DRAINAGE OF STOMACH

SMALL INTESTINE OVERVIEW

SECTION THROUGH DUODENUM

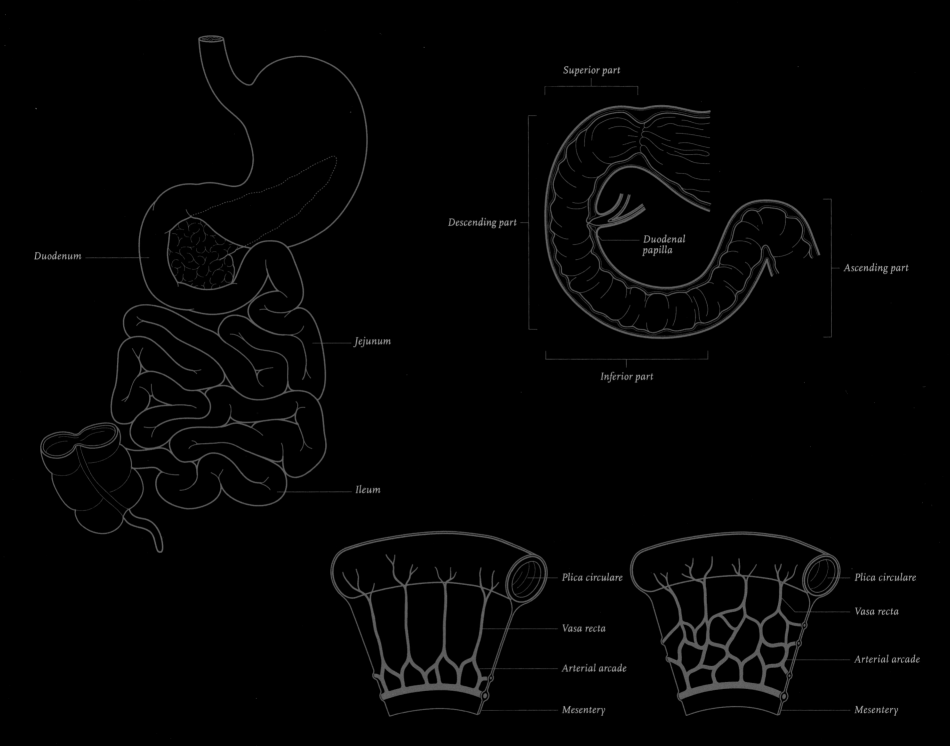

Duodenum

Jejunum

Ileum

Superior part

Descending part

Duodenal
papilla

Ascending part

Inferior part

Plica circulare

Vasa recta

Arterial arcade

Mesentery

Plica circulare

Vasa recta

Arterial arcade

Mesentery

JEJUNUM

ILEUM

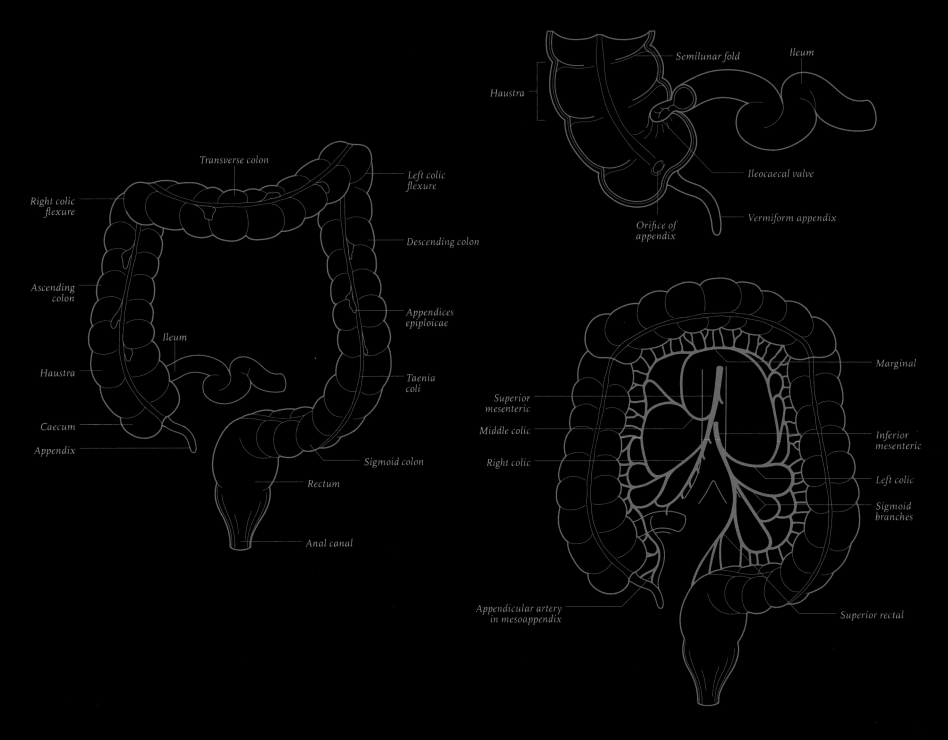

Transverse colon

Left colic
flexure

Right colic
flexure

Descending colon

Ascending
colon

Appendices
epiploicae

Ileum

Taenia
coli

Haustra

Caecum

Appendix

Sigmoid colon

Rectum

Anal canal

Semilunar fold

Ileum

Haustra

Ileocaecal valve

Orifice of
appendix

Vermiform appendix

Superior
mesenteric

Marginal

Middle colic

Inferior
mesenteric

Right colic

Left colic

Sigmoid
branches

Appendicular artery
in mesoappendix

Superior rectal

ARTERIES OF LARGE INTESTINE

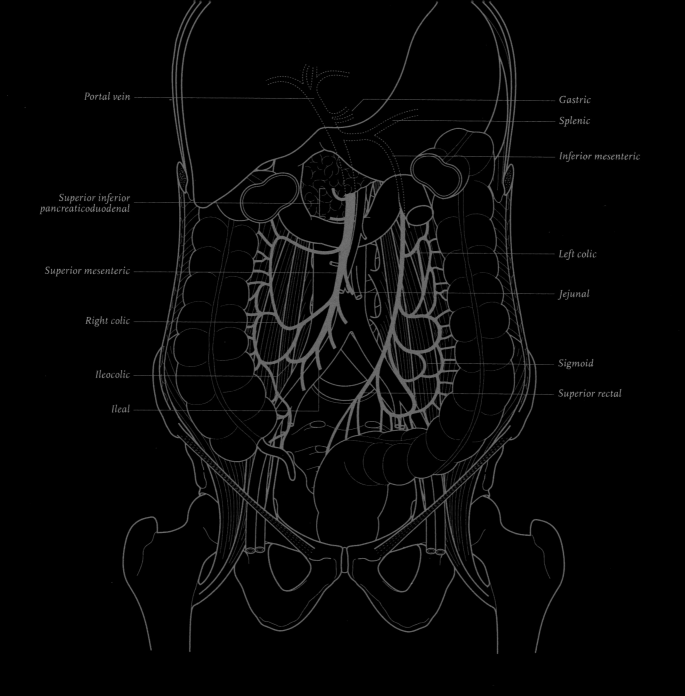

Portal vein

Superior inferior
pancreaticoduodenal

Superior mesenteric

Right colic

Ileocolic

Ileal

Gastric

Splenic

Inferior mesenteric

Left colic

Jejunal

Sigmoid

Superior rectal

ANTERIOR VIEW OF LIVER

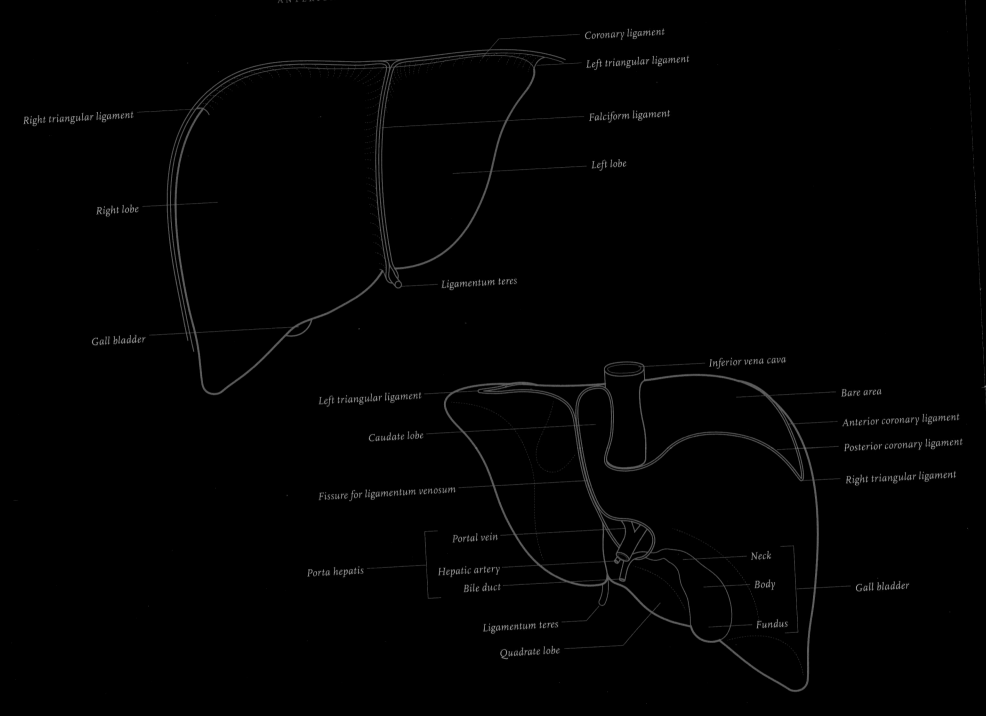

Coronary ligament

Left triangular ligament

Right triangular ligament

Falciform ligament

Left lobe

Right lobe

Ligamentum teres

Gall bladder

Inferior vena cava

Left triangular ligament

Bare area

Caudate lobe

Anterior coronary ligament

Posterior coronary ligament

Right triangular ligament

Fissure for ligamentum venosum

Portal vein

Neck

Porta hepatis

Hepatic artery

Body

Gall bladder

Bile duct

Ligamentum teres

Fundus

Quadrate lobe

POSTERIOR VIEW OF LIVER

HEPATIC BLOOD SUPPLY & BILE VESSELS

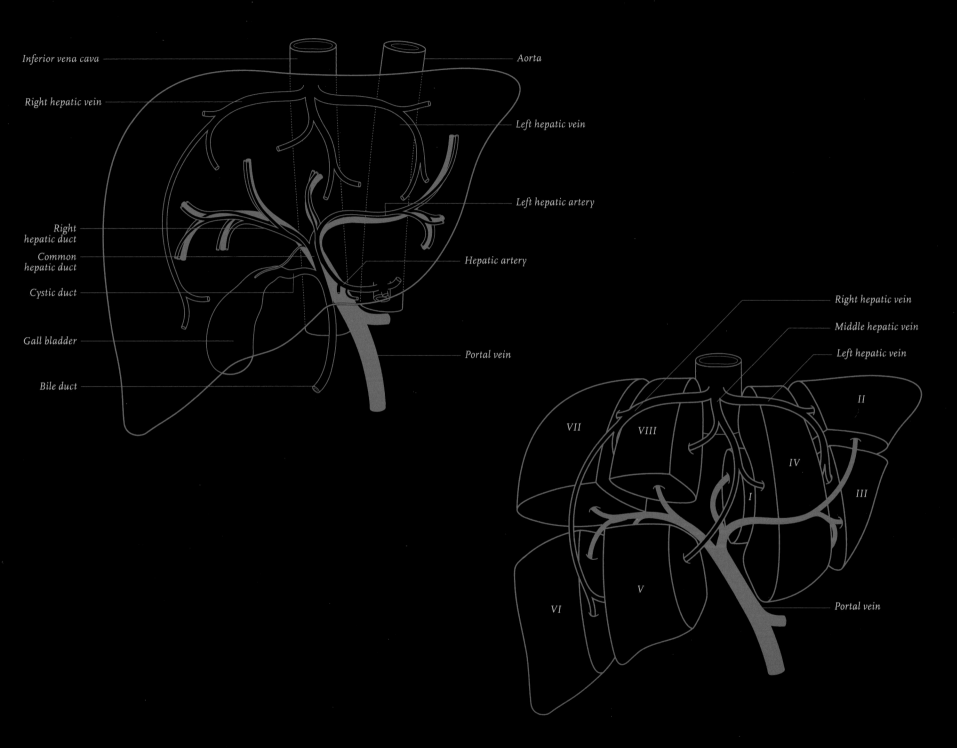

Inferior vena cava

Right hepatic vein

Right
hepatic duct

Common
hepatic duct

Cystic duct

Gall bladder

Bile duct

Aorta

Left hepatic vein

Left hepatic artery

Hepatic artery

Portal vein

Right hepatic vein

Middle hepatic vein

Left hepatic vein

II

VII

VIII

IV

I

III

V

VI

Portal vein

HEPATIC SEGMENTS

THE PANCREAS, SPLEEN & KIDNEYS

The pancreas, spleen, kidneys and ureters are retroperitoneal, because they lie on the posterior abdominal wall together with the abdominal aorta and inferior vena cava behind the peritoneum.

The pancreas lies posterior to the stomach with its head in the curve of the duodenum, and its tail pointing towards the hilum of the spleen. It is composed of glandular tissue that manufactures digestive enzymes, which drain into the pancreatic duct to be eventually secreted into the duodenum. It also produces insulin and glucagon to regulate blood glucose levels. Between the uncinate process and the neck lie the superior mesenteric vessels. These contribute pancreaticoduodenal branches, which supply the pancreas, as do branches from the splenic arteries.

The spleen is supplied by the splenic branch of the coeliac artery. The splenic vein joins the superior mesenteric vein to form the portal vein. It resides in the left hypochondrium of the abdomen against the diaphragm and is related to ribs 9–11. It has an immunological function, processing incoming blood.

The kidneys filter a vast amount of blood every minute. They therefore have arterial supply direct from the abdominal aorta (renal arteries) and venous drainage by the renal veins into the inferior vena cava. These paired organs lie on either side of the lumbar vertebral column, with the left slightly higher than the right. They are encapsulated by perirenal fat contained within the renal fascia to protect them against impact forces. Right and left adrenal glands rest on the upper pole on the right kidney and medial border on the left kidney outside the renal capsules. Filtration occurs in the cortex and inner medulla of the kidney, which is encased in a fibrous capsule. Filtered blood plasma drains into the minor and major calyces, where it collects in the renal pelvis to be drained by the ureter as urine. The tubular ureters run inferiorly anterior to the tips of the transverse processes of the lumbar vertebrae and psoas major. They cross anterior to the bifurcation of the common iliac artery and vein at the pelvic brim, where they turn medially to enter the posteroinferior aspect of the bladder.

The autonomic nervous system is concerned with the innervation of smooth muscle and glands. It comprises two opposite systems: sympathetic and parasympathetic innervation. Parasympathetic nerve supply to the abdominal viscera is via the vagus nerve (CN X) (meaning wandering, as it travels a long way from the brain to supply the abdominal viscera) and pelvic splanchnic nerves. Parasympathetic division controls the restful state, encouraging digestion and glandular secretion. Sympathetic innervation triggers the 'fight or flight' response, increasing heart rate and blood flow to muscles, thereby opposing restful digestive functions. Neurons from the sympathetic chain and the splanchnic nerves synapse in the ganglia situated around major blood vessels before going on to innervate the target organs.

ABDOMINAL RETROPERITONEAL STRUCTURES

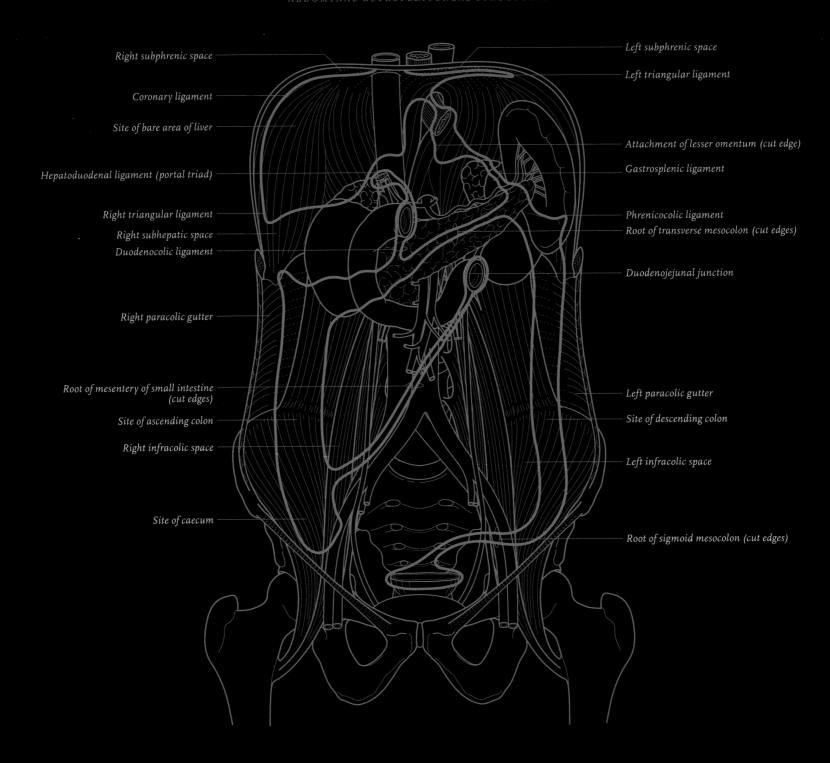

Right subphrenic space

Coronary ligament

Site of bare area of liver

Hepatoduodenal ligament (portal triad)

Right triangular ligament

Right subhepatic space

Duodenocolic ligament

Right paracolic gutter

Root of mesentery of small intestine
(cut edges)

Site of ascending colon

Right infracolic space

Site of caecum

Left subphrenic space

Left triangular ligament

Attachment of lesser omentum (cut edge)

Gastrosplenic ligament

Phrenicocolic ligament

Root of transverse mesocolon (cut edges)

Duodenojejunal junction

Left paracolic gutter

Site of descending colon

Left infracolic space

Root of sigmoid mesocolon (cut edges)

SECTION THROUGH PANCREAS & BILE DUCT

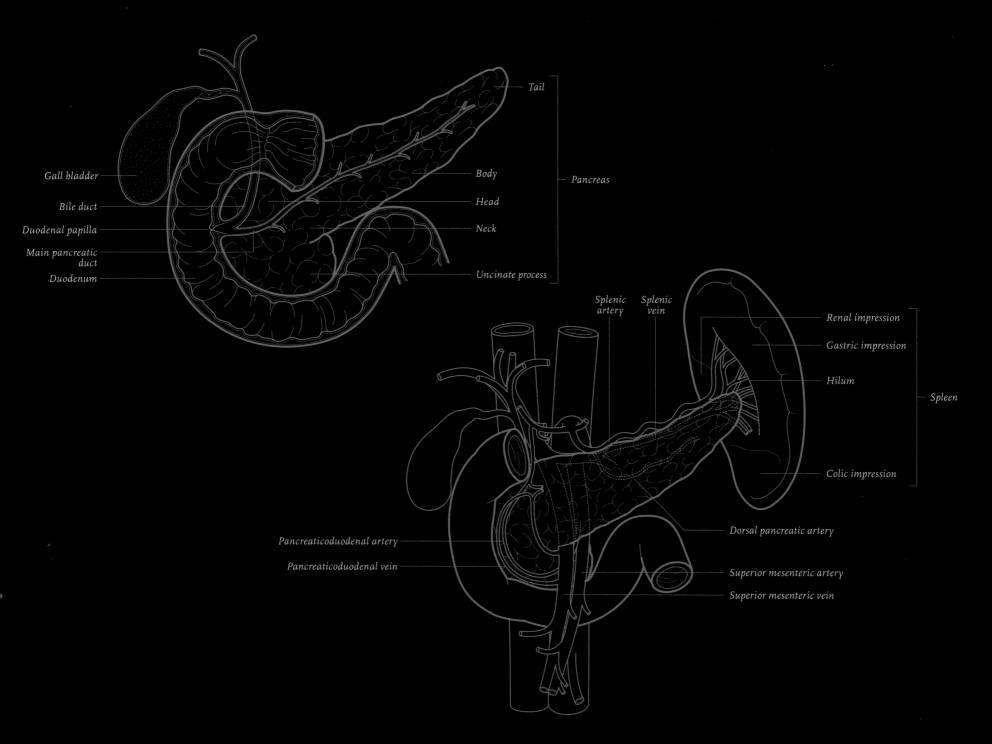

Tail

Gall bladder

Body — Pancreas

Bile duct

Head

Duodenal papilla

Neck

Main pancreatic
duct

Duodenum

Uncinate process

Splenic
artery

Splenic
vein

Renal impression

Gastric impression

Hilum

Spleen

Colic impression

Pancreaticoduodenal artery

Pancreaticoduodenal vein

Dorsal pancreatic artery

Superior mesenteric artery

Superior mesenteric vein

BLOOD SUPPLY TO PANCREAS & SPLEEN

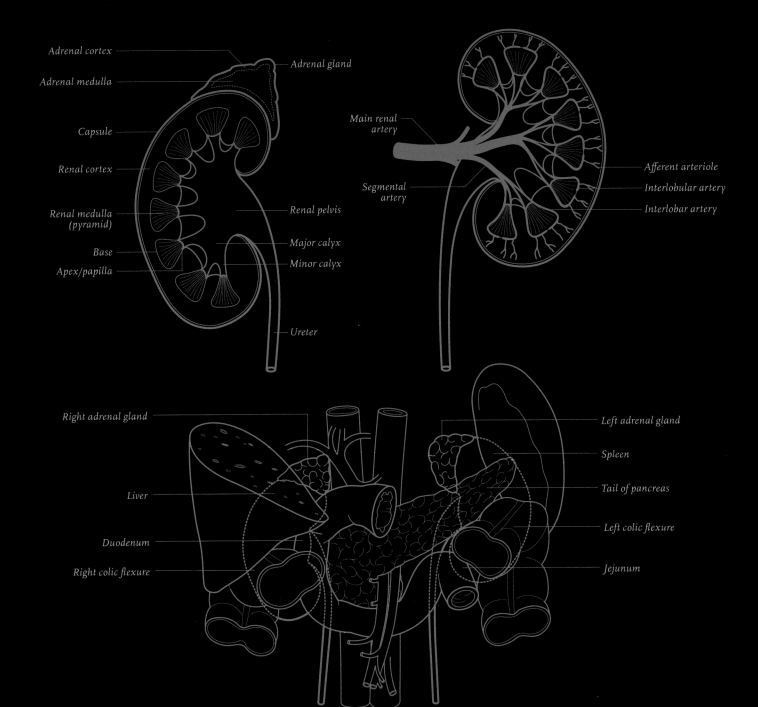

CORONAL SECTION OF RIGHT KIDNEY

ARTERIES OF LEFT KIDNEY

Adrenal cortex

Adrenal medulla

Capsule

Renal cortex

Renal medulla
(pyramid)

Base

Apex/papilla

Adrenal gland

Renal pelvis

Major calyx

Minor calyx

Ureter

Main renal
artery

Segmental
artery

Afferent arteriole

Interlobular artery

Interlobar artery

Right adrenal gland

Liver

Duodenum

Right colic flexure

Left adrenal gland

Spleen

Tail of pancreas

Left colic flexure

Jejunum

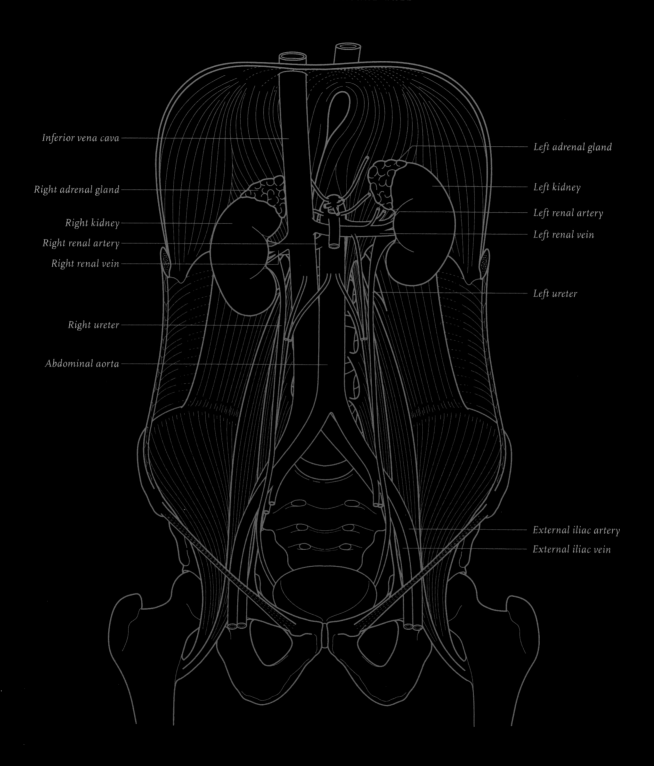

Inferior vena cava

Right adrenal gland

Right kidney

Right renal artery

Right renal vein

Right ureter

Abdominal aorta

Left adrenal gland

Left kidney

Left renal artery

Left renal vein

Left ureter

External iliac artery

External iliac vein

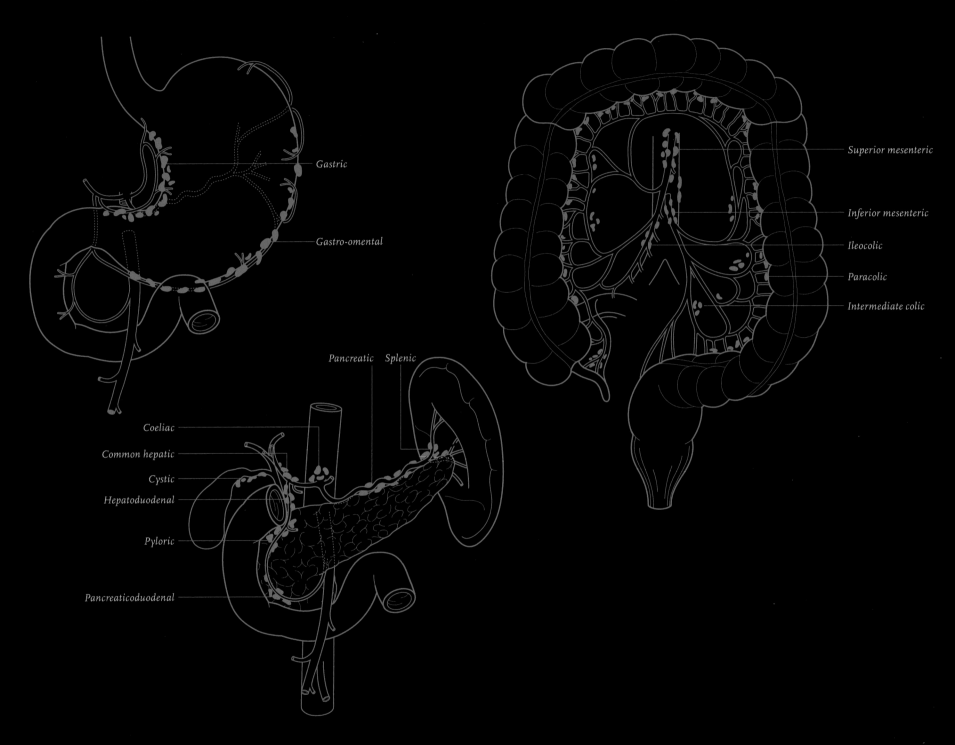

Gastric

Gastro-omental

Superior mesenteric

Inferior mesenteric

Ileocolic

Paracolic

Intermediate colic

Pancreatic   Splenic

Coeliac

Common hepatic

Cystic

Hepatoduodenal

Pyloric

Pancreaticoduodenal

LYMPH NODES OF PANCREAS

ABDOMINAL AUTONOMIC NERVE SUPPLY

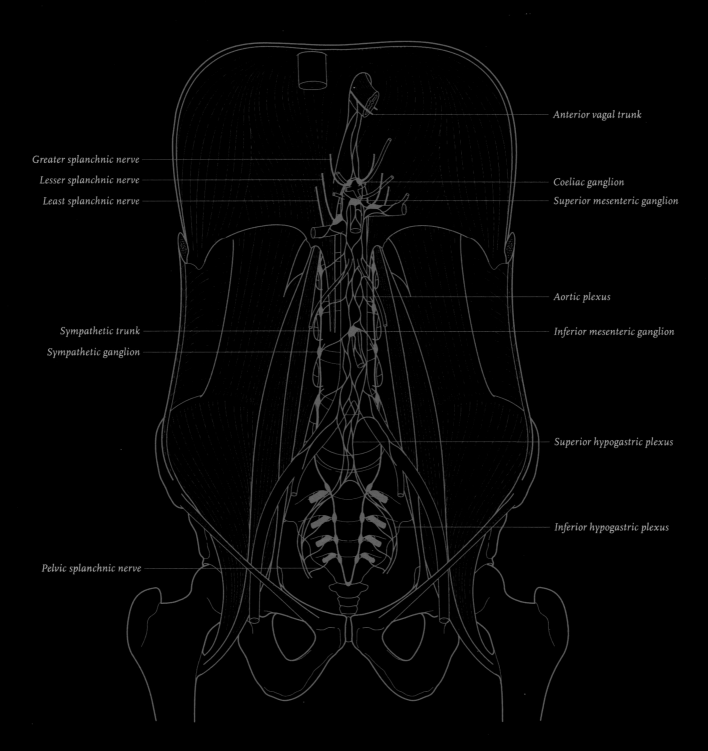

Anterior vagal trunk

Greater splanchnic nerve

Lesser splanchnic nerve

Least splanchnic nerve

Coeliac ganglion

Superior mesenteric ganglion

Aortic plexus

Sympathetic trunk

Inferior mesenteric ganglion

Sympathetic ganglion

Superior hypogastric plexus

Inferior hypogastric plexus

Pelvic splanchnic nerve

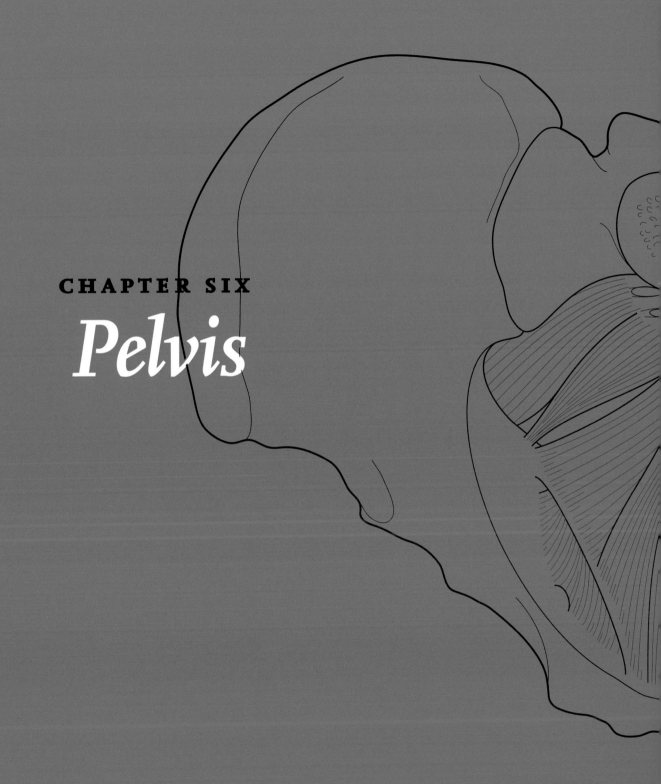

CHAPTER SIX
Pelvis

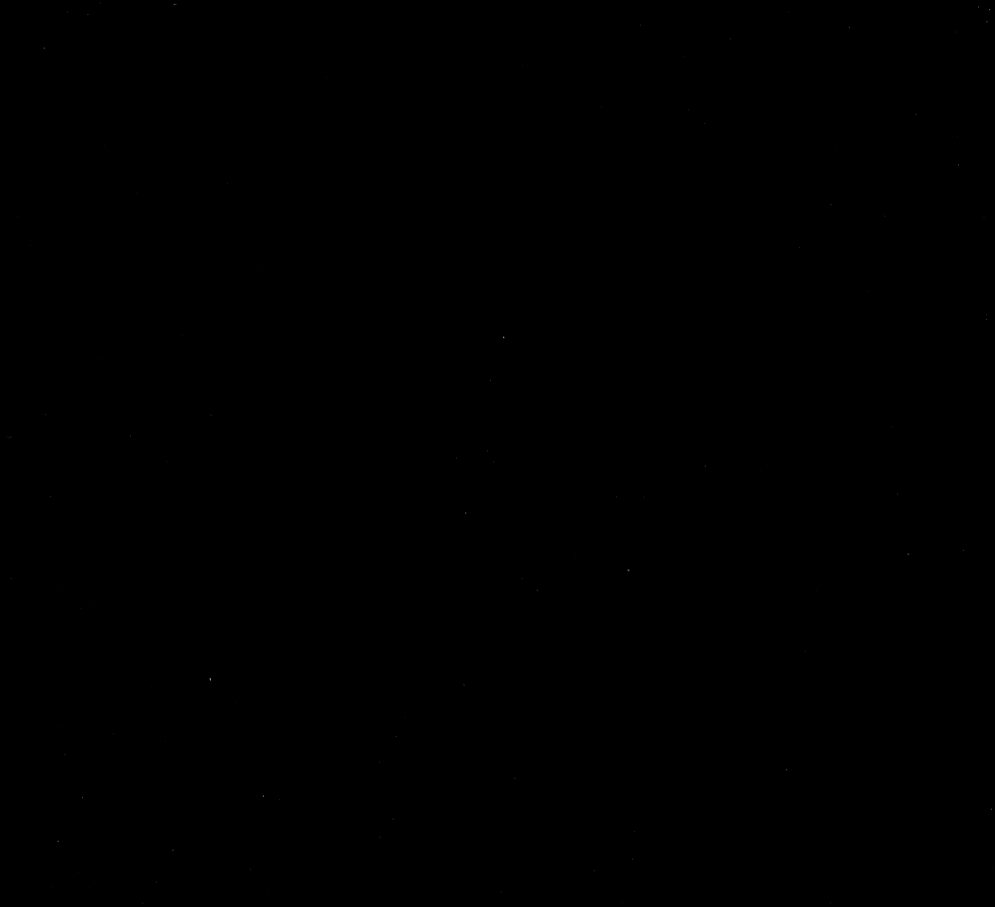

THE BONES & MUSCLES

Two pelvic bones, along with the sacrum and the coccyx, constitute the pelvis. Each pelvic bone consists of three fused bones, the ilium, ischium and pubis that converge in the acetabulum. The two pelvic bones fuse in the midline at the cartilaginous symphysis pubis joint, and posteriorly with the sacrum, forming two synovial sacroiliac joints. Structurally, the sacrum acts as a 'keystone' to transfer the weight of the upper body and torso effectively through to the lower limb.

The pelvic inlet is the entrance to the pelvic cavity and is marked by the sacral promontory, following around the arcuate line and pelvic brim. The shape of this varies from heart-shaped in males to wider and more circular in females. Two other distinctions between the pelvises of each of the sexes are the subpubic angle and the distance between the ischial spines, both being greater in the female. All of these differences serve to facilitate childbirth in females.

Two ligaments on the pelvic wall (sacrotuberous, sacrospinous) define the apertures known as the greater and lesser sciatic foramina. Other than the bones of the pelvis below the inlet, two muscles also contribute to the wall: obturator internus and piriformis, both lateral rotators of the hip joint.

The remaining muscles form the pelvic floor (comprising the levator ani and coccygeus muscles), which separates the pelvic cavity from the perineum below. Collectively named the pelvic diaphragm, its bowl-like structure supports the pelvic viscera. The four component muscles of levator ani form sling-like muscle bands around the orifices and together work with intra-abdominal pressure to assist micturition, defaecation and childbirth.

The pelvic outlet is diamond-shaped and can be divided by a line between the ischial tuberosities into urogenital and anal triangles.

The urogenital triangle contains the urethral and vaginal orifices, clitoris, and related structures in the female, and penis, scrotum and related structures in the male. These structures are supported by the perineal membrane. Erectile tissue of the clitoris and penis is clothed in bulbospongiosus and ischiocavernosus muscles.

The anal triangle contains the anal orifice, which is enclosed by the external anal sphincter. Between its floor, formed by levator ani, and the skin is the fat-filled ischioanal fossa.

Muscles converge in a central perineal body, which is essential for supporting the pelvic viscera and is stabilised by the transverse perineal muscle.

ANTERIOR PELVIS (MALE)

ANTERIOR PELVIS (FEMALE)

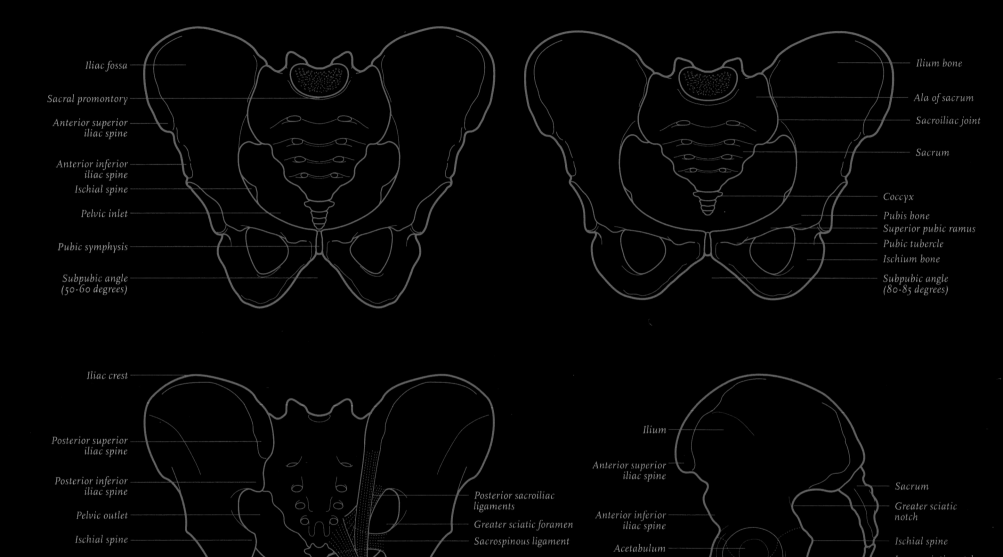

Iliac fossa

Sacral promontory

Anterior superior
iliac spine

Anterior inferior
iliac spine

Ischial spine

Pelvic inlet

Pubic symphysis

Subpubic angle
(50-60 degrees)

Ilium bone

Ala of sacrum

Sacroiliac joint

Sacrum

Coccyx

Pubis bone
Superior pubic ramus
Pubic tubercle
Ischium bone

Subpubic angle
(80-85 degrees)

Iliac crest

Posterior superior
iliac spine

Posterior inferior
iliac spine

Pelvic outlet

Ischial spine

Obturator foramen

Ischial tuberosity

Posterior sacroiliac
ligaments

Greater sciatic foramen

Sacrospinous ligament

Lesser sciatic foramen

Sacrotuberous ligament

Ilium

Anterior superior
iliac spine

Anterior inferior
iliac spine

Acetabulum

Pubis

Sacrum

Greater sciatic
notch

Ischial spine

Lesser sciatic notch
Coccyx

Ischial tuberosity

Ischium

POSTERIOR PELVIS

LATERAL PELVIS

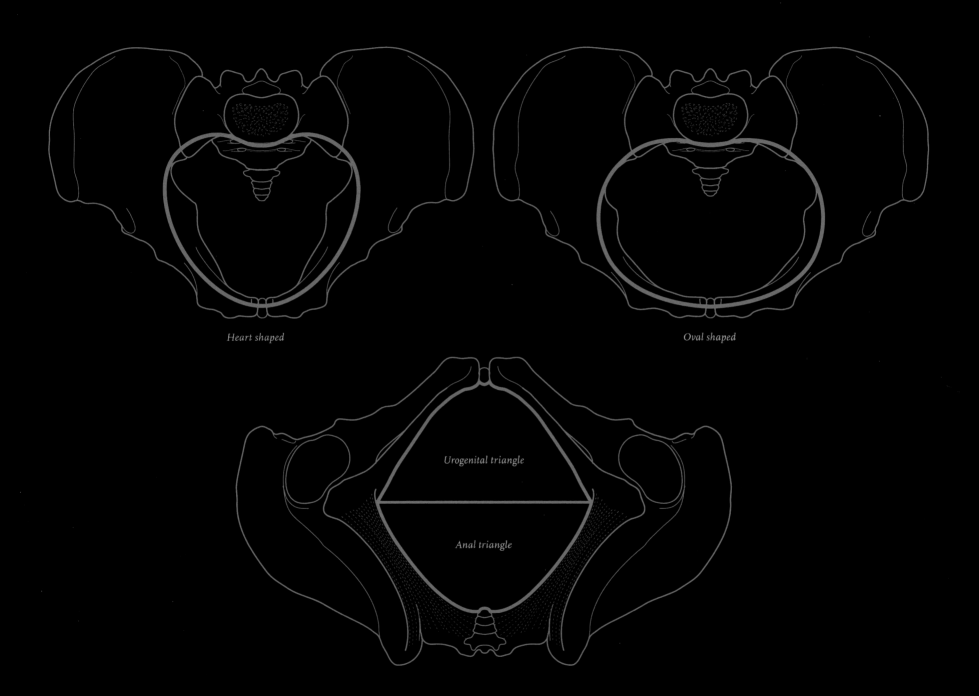

Heart shaped

Oval shaped

Urogenital triangle

Anal triangle

PELVIC OUTLET WITH BOUNDARIES OF PERINEUM

CORONAL VIEW OF UROGENITAL TRIANGLE

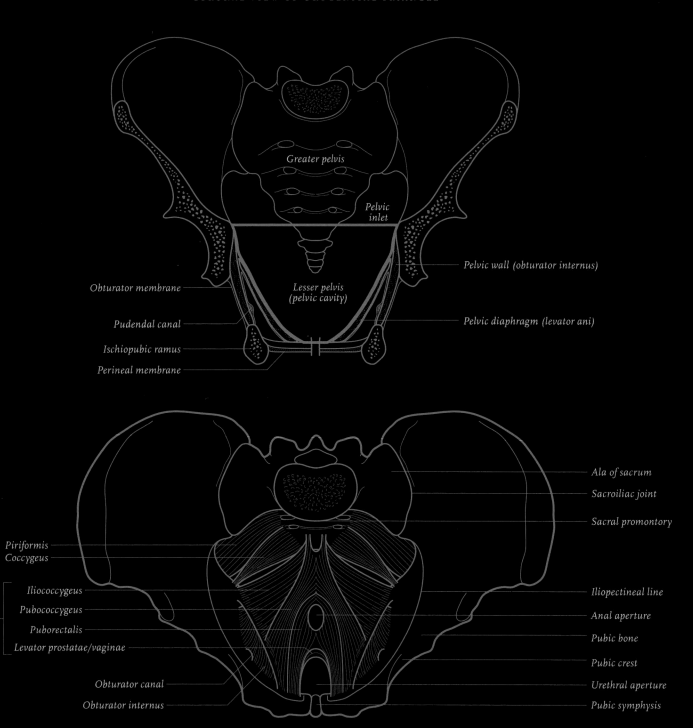

Greater pelvis

Pelvic inlet

Pelvic wall (obturator internus)

Obturator membrane

Lesser pelvis (pelvic cavity)

Pudendal canal

Pelvic diaphragm (levator ani)

Ischiopubic ramus

Perineal membrane

Ala of sacrum

Sacroiliac joint

Sacral promontory

Piriformis
Coccygeus

Iliococcygeus

Iliopectineal line

Pubococcygeus

Anal aperture

Levator ani

Puborectalis

Pubic bone

Levator prostatae/vaginae

Pubic crest

Obturator canal

Urethral aperture

Obturator internus

Pubic symphysis

SUPERIOR VIEW OF PELVIC MUSCLES

142

PERINEUM (FEMALE)

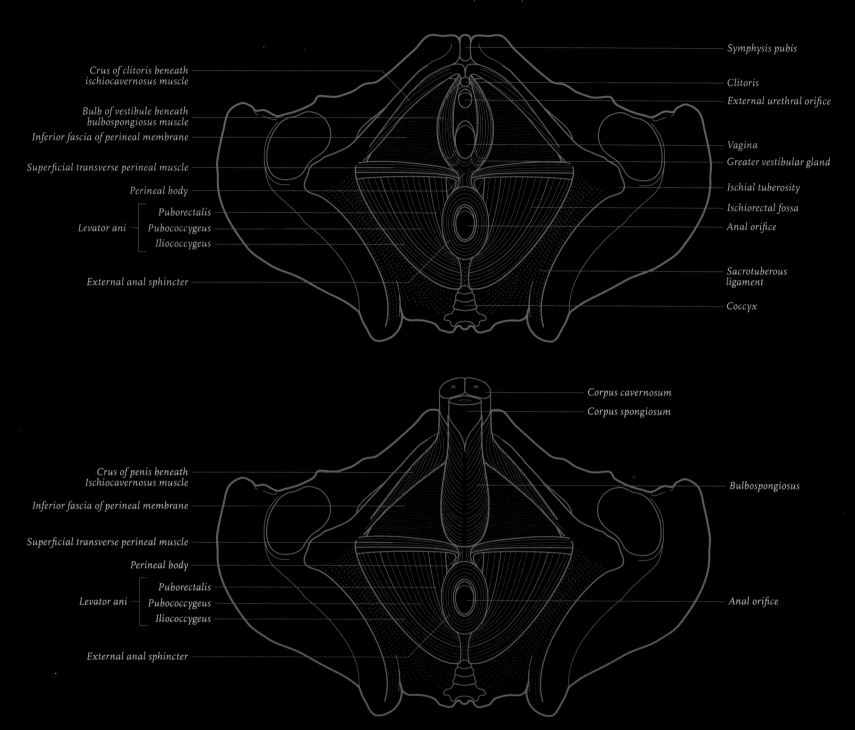

Crus of clitoris beneath
ischiocavernosus muscle

Bulb of vestibule beneath
bulbospongiosus muscle

Inferior fascia of perineal membrane

Superficial transverse perineal muscle

Perineal body

Puborectalis
Levator ani — Pubococcygeus
Iliococcygeus

External anal sphincter

Symphysis pubis

Clitoris

External urethral orifice

Vagina

Greater vestibular gland

Ischial tuberosity

Ischiorectal fossa

Anal orifice

Sacrotuberous
ligament

Coccyx

Crus of penis beneath
Ischiocavernosus muscle

Inferior fascia of perineal membrane

Superficial transverse perineal muscle

Perineal body

Puborectalis
Levator ani — Pubococcygeus
Iliococcygeus

External anal sphincter

Corpus cavernosum

Corpus spongiosum

Bulbospongiosus

Anal orifice

PERINEUM (MALE)

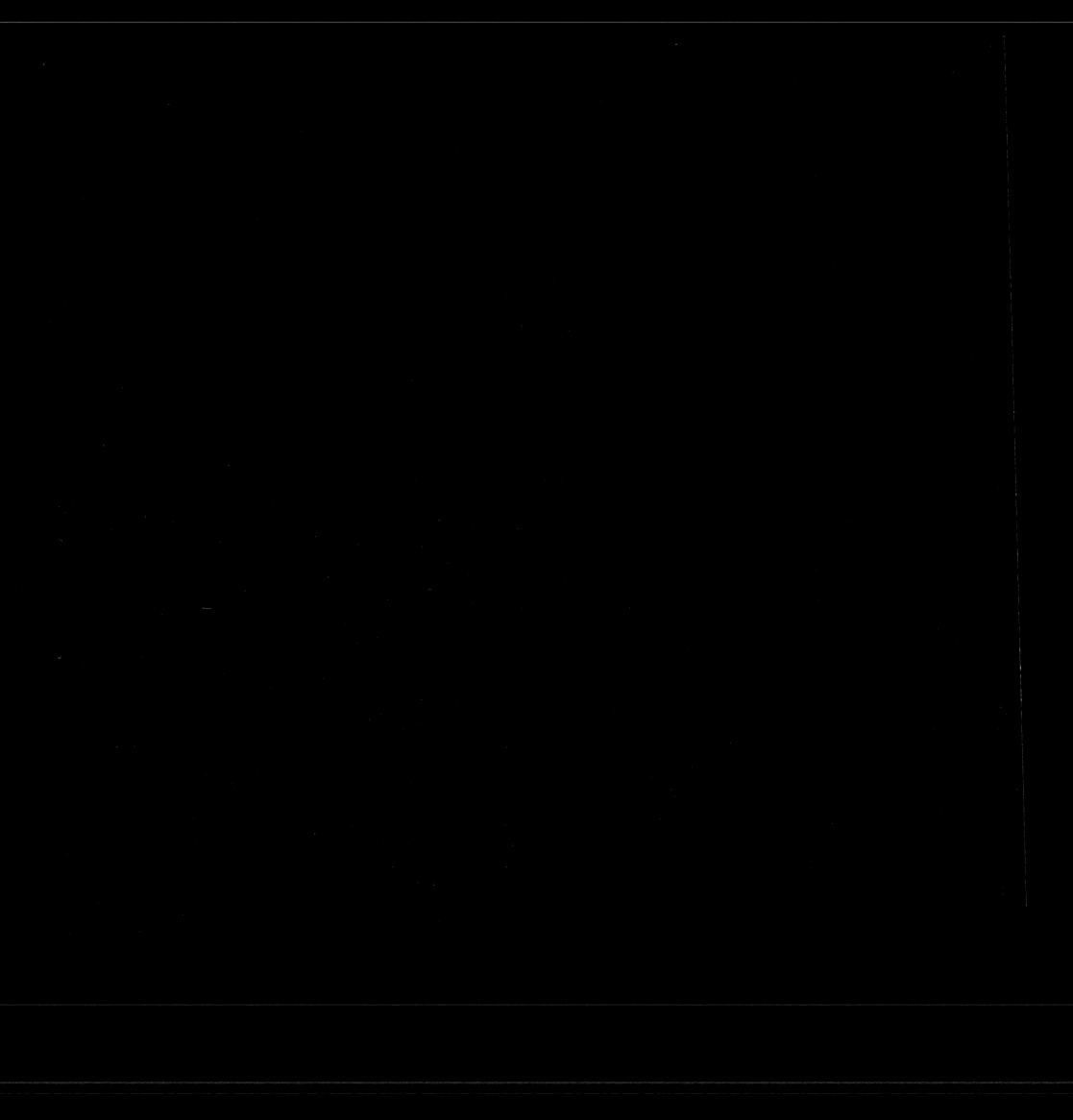

THE REPRODUCTIVE ORGANS

The peritoneal lining of the abdominal cavity covers the structures of the pelvis and creates pouches between the pelvic viscera. The rectovesical pouch is located between the bladder and the rectum in the male. In the female there are the vesicouterine pouch between the bladder and uterus and the rectouterine pouch between the rectum and uterus.

The ovary serves as the primary organ of the female reproductive system by producing the germ cells, the ova. These are collected on their monthly release from the ovary by the finger-like fimbriae and guided down the fallopian tubes to the uterine cavity. The ovary, like the testis, descends from the posterior abdominal wall in fetal development to lie suspended by the suspensory ligament of the ovary containing the ovarian artery and vein (branches of the abdominal aorta and inferior vena cava/left renal vein respectively). It is moored to the uterus by the ovarian ligament, which is clothed, together with the fundus and body of the uterus and the fallopian tubes, by a layer of peritoneum termed the broad ligament, which has various portions attributed with names according to their position. The uterus, composed of smooth muscle, serves as a site for implantation of the embryo; its rich endothelium nourishing the growth of the fetus. It is usually anteflexed (bent) and anteverted (tilted) so its body curves superiorly over the bladder.

The fibromuscular vagina joins the uterus at its inferior extremity in an area called the cervix. Its central aperture (external os) is where the sperm enters the uterine cavity for fertilisation of the ovum, and it subsequently relaxes in childbirth. The vagina then acts as a birth canal for the fetus.

The primary organs of the male reproductive system that produce the germ cells are the testes. These are suspended in a sac of skin and covering of the spermatic cord, the scrotum, outside the body cavity to maintain the effective production of sperm at below body temperature. A complex series of venous blood vessels (the pampiniform plexus of veins) provide a countercurrent effect to cool the arterial blood from the testicular artery to maintain this temperature. Sperm produced in the testes travel in the seminiferous tubules to the epididymis, where they are stored and recycled if not used. With stimulus, sperm are transmitted in the smooth-muscle-walled tube, the ductus deferens, up through the inguinal canal in the anterior abdominal wall into the abdominal cavity, and subsequently terminate in the prostatic urethra. Here, fluid from the seminal vesicles, which lie on the posterior inferior surface of the bladder, together with prostatic secretions, joins the mature sperm to form semen. The bulbourethral glands secrete into the spongy urethra where the semen travels through the penis.

The penis consists of three compartments: two corpus cavernosa chambers divided by a septum, sitting above the corpus spongiosum, which surrounds the urethra. The erectile tissue in these compartments is held within a fibrous tunica albuginea to prevent overexpansion. With stimulus, blood supply through the cavernosus artery is increased, and the cavernosal sinuses fill with blood. Blood drainage is reduced as the erectile tissue compresses the dorsal veins by pressing them against the capsule.

Blood supply to the pelvic organs is via branches of the internal iliac artery and drainage by branches of the internal iliac vein. The pudendal nerve supplies the majority of the muscles in the perineum with sympathetic and parasympathetic innervation originating from the superior and inferior hypogastric plexuses.

SAGITTAL SECTION THROUGH FEMALE PELVIS

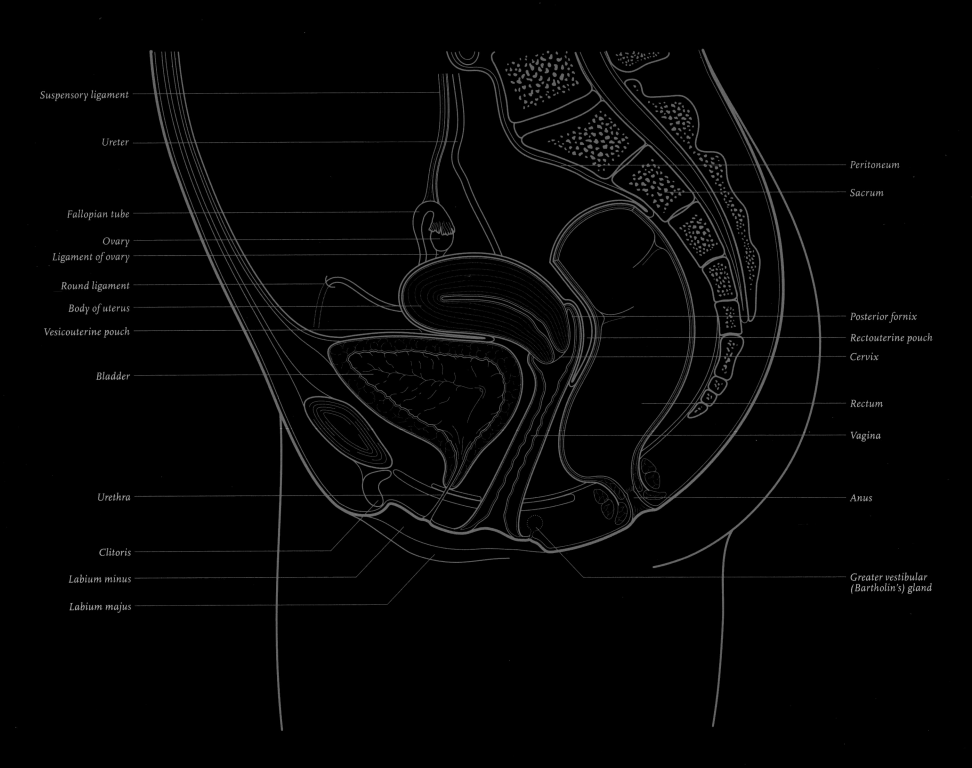

Suspensory ligament

Ureter

Fallopian tube

Ovary

Ligament of ovary

Round ligament

Body of uterus

Vesicouterine pouch

Bladder

Urethra

Clitoris

Labium minus

Labium majus

Peritoneum

Sacrum

Posterior fornix

Rectouterine pouch

Cervix

Rectum

Vagina

Anus

Greater vestibular
(Bartholin's) gland

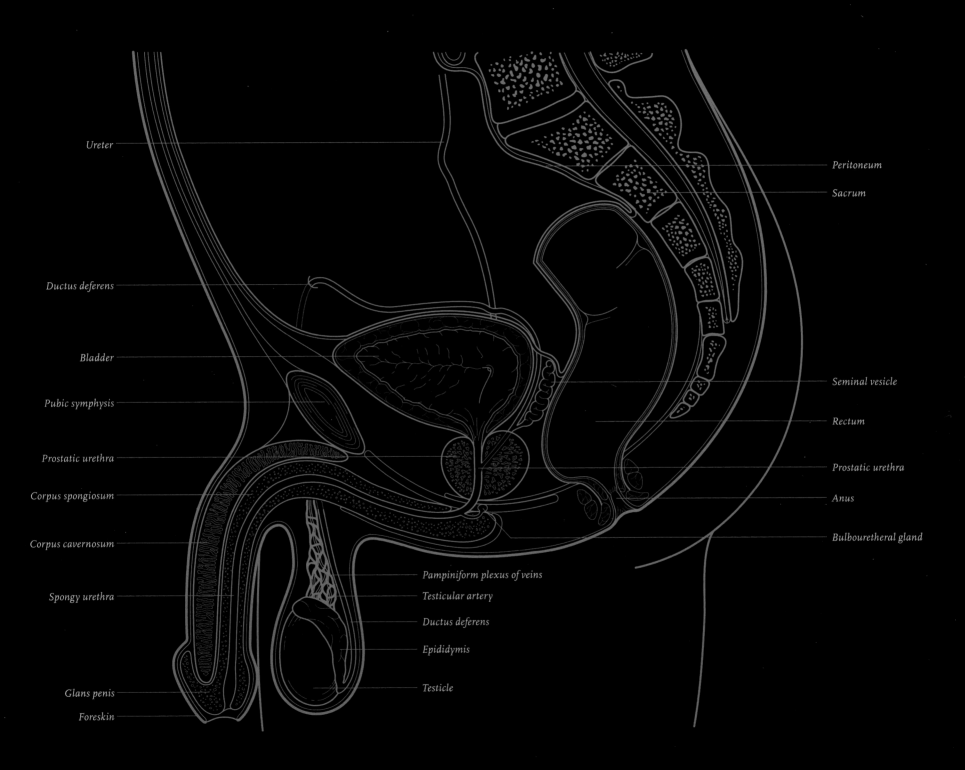

Ureter

Peritoneum

Sacrum

Ductus deferens

Bladder

Seminal vesicle

Pubic symphysis

Rectum

Prostatic urethra

Prostatic urethra

Corpus spongiosum

Anus

Corpus cavernosum

Bulbouretheral gland

Pampiniform plexus of veins

Spongy urethra

Testicular artery

Ductus deferens

Epididymis

Glans penis

Testicle

Foreskin

ANTERIOR VIEW OF UTERUS & VAGINA

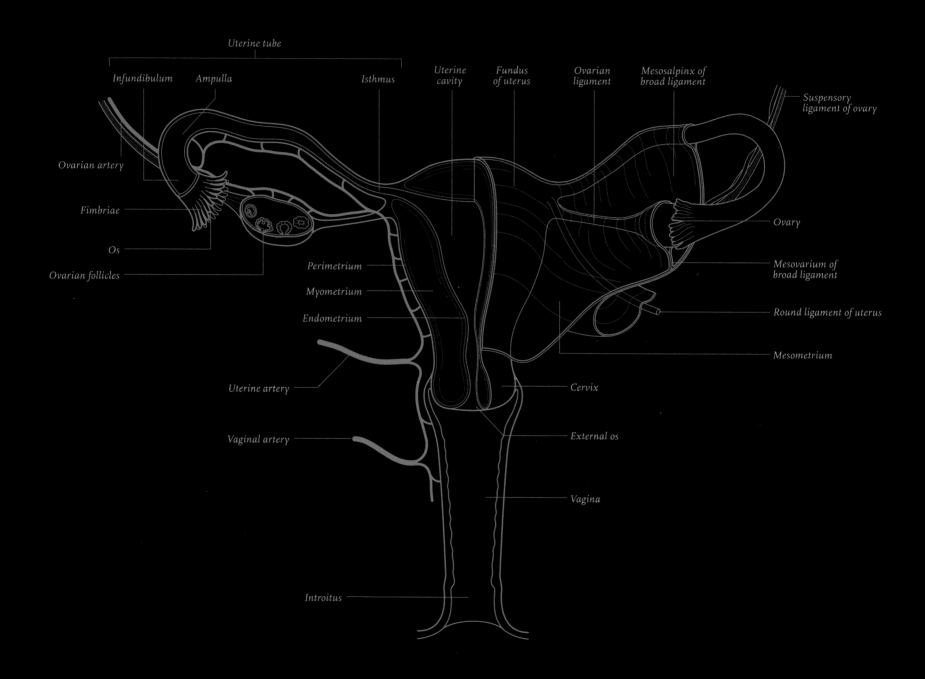

Uterine tube

Infundibulum   Ampulla   Isthmus   Uterine cavity   Fundus of uterus   Ovarian ligament   Mesosalpinx of broad ligament   Suspensory ligament of ovary

Ovarian artery

Fimbriae

Os   Ovary

Ovarian follicles   Mesovarium of broad ligament

Perimetrium

Myometrium   Round ligament of uterus

Endometrium   Mesometrium

Uterine artery   Cervix

Vaginal artery   External os

Vagina

Introitus

SECTION THROUGH PENIS

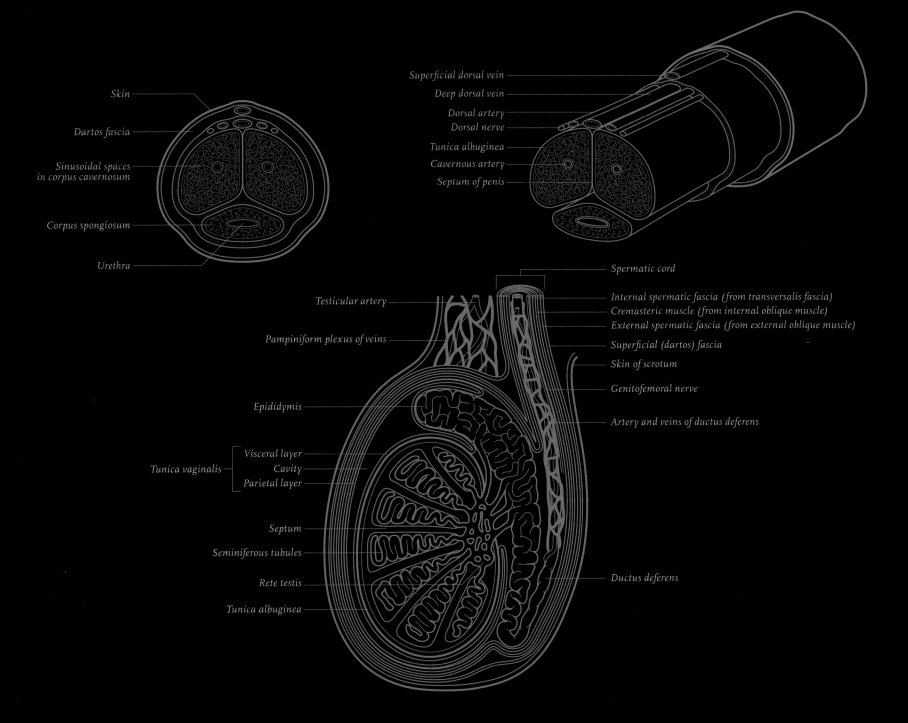

Skin

Dartos fascia

Sinusoidal spaces
in corpus cavernosum

Corpus spongiosum

Urethra

Superficial dorsal vein

Deep dorsal vein

Dorsal artery

Dorsal nerve

Tunica albuginea

Cavernous artery

Septum of penis

Spermatic cord

Internal spermatic fascia (from transversalis fascia)

Cremasteric muscle (from internal oblique muscle)

External spermatic fascia (from external oblique muscle)

Superficial (dartos) fascia

Skin of scrotum

Genitofemoral nerve

Artery and veins of ductus deferens

Testicular artery

Pampiniform plexus of veins

Epididymis

Tunica vaginalis

Visceral layer

Cavity

Parietal layer

Septum

Seminiferous tubules

Rete testis

Tunica albuginea

Ductus deferens

SAGITTAL VIEW OF TESTIS

THE BLADDER & RECTUM

The urinary bladder lies posterior to the pubic symphysis and is covered superiorly by peritoneum. It has muscular walls (the detrusor muscle) lined with transitional epithelium, which is a membrane that can withstand the toxicity of urine, and undergo a high degree of stretching. When the bladder is distended, it rises above the pubic symphysis.

The ureters are also lined with transitional epithelium, and transmit the urine produced by the kidneys to their junction at the base of the bladder. The mucosal area between the two ureteral orifices and the urethral orifice is called the trigone. An internal sphincter formed of smooth muscle lies at the urethral opening and relaxes when the bladder is full.

In males, the presence of the prostate gland beneath the bladder neck creates a section of the urethra known as the prostatic urethra. This area receives the openings of the ducts that contribute to the seminal fluid. Distal to the prostatic urethra is the membranous urethra at the level of the perineal membrane, and the spongy urethra within the corpus spongiosum of the penis.

In females, the short urethra of the bladder lies anterior to the vagina and is surrounded by a urethral sphincter on the perineal membrane. The bladder is supplied by the superior and inferior vesical arteries, branches of the internal iliac artery. Venous drainage is via a venous plexus at the base of the bladder (and additionally in males by the prostatic venous plexus). Parasympathetic innervation for micturition is via the pelvic splanchnic nerves, and sympathetics run from the hypogastric plexus.

The rectum is a continuation of the sigmoid colon and begins around the third sacral vertebra. It continues forwards at the coccyx and widens as the rectal ampulla, before passing backwards through the pelvic diaphragm around puborectalis. As it narrows inferiorly, it becomes the anal canal. Folds of mucosa called anal columns and depressions called anal sinuses form a ring at a location termed the pectinate line. This line marks a transition between blood supply (superior rectal arteries and vein above and inferior below), and innervation (inferior hypogastric plexus and pelvic splanchnic nerves above and inferior rectal nerves from the pudendal nerve sensitive to pain, touch and temperature below the line).

The anal orifice is surrounded by both internal and external sphincter muscles. The internal sphincter is involuntary (pelvic splanchnic nerves), and the external sphincter is under voluntary control from the inferior rectal nerve.

CORONAL SECTION THROUGH MALE URINARY BLADDER

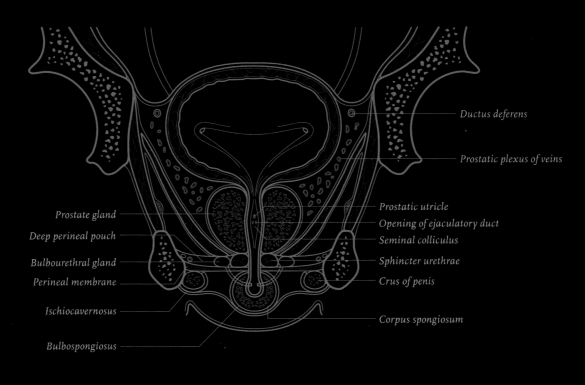

Ductus deferens

Prostatic plexus of veins

Prostate gland

Prostatic utricle

Deep perineal pouch

Opening of ejaculatory duct

Seminal colliculus

Bulbourethral gland

Sphincter urethrae

Perineal membrane

Crus of penis

Ischiocavernosus

Corpus spongiosum

Bulbospongiosus

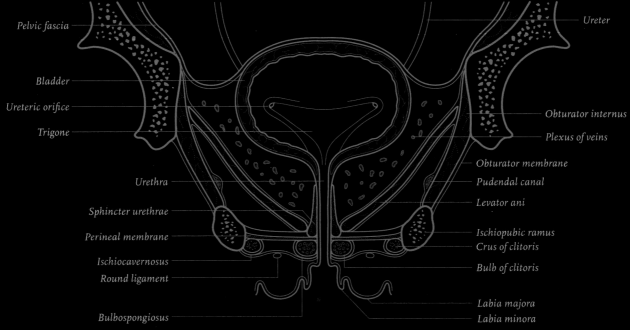

Pelvic fascia

Ureter

Bladder

Ureteric orifice

Obturator internus

Trigone

Plexus of veins

Obturator membrane

Urethra

Pudendal canal

Sphincter urethrae

Levator ani

Perineal membrane

Ischiopubic ramus

Crus of clitoris

Ischiocavernosus

Bulb of clitoris

Round ligament

Labia majora

Bulbospongiosus

Labia minora

CORONAL SECTION THROUGH FEMALE URINARY BLADDER

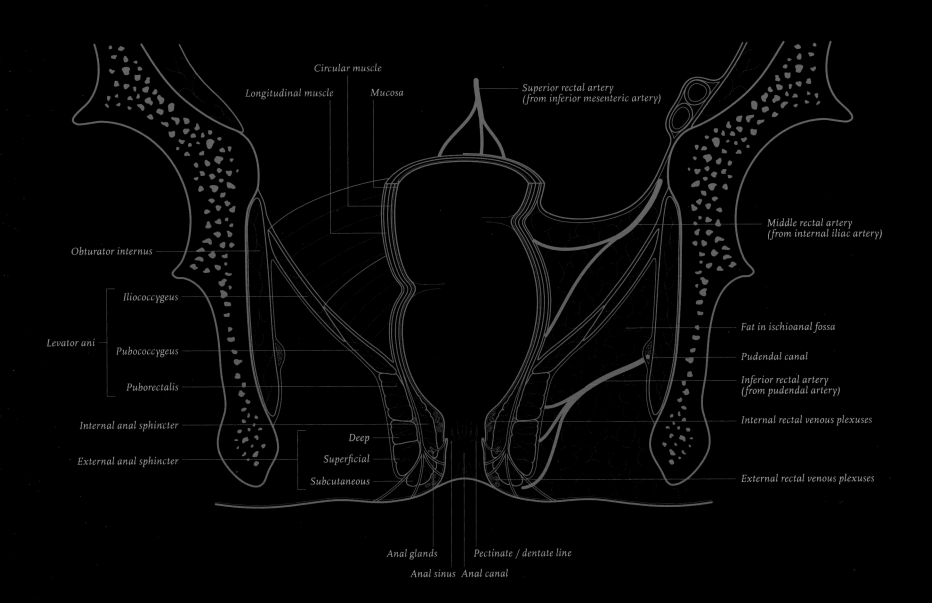

Circular muscle

Longitudinal muscle

Mucosa

Superior rectal artery
(from inferior mesenteric artery)

Obturator internus

Iliococcygeus

Levator ani

Pubococcygeus

Puborectalis

Internal anal sphincter

External anal sphincter

Middle rectal artery
(from internal iliac artery)

Fat in ischioanal fossa

Pudendal canal

Inferior rectal artery
(from pudendal artery)

Internal rectal venous plexuses

External rectal venous plexuses

Deep

Superficial

Subcutaneous

Anal glands

Pectinate / dentate line

Anal sinus Anal canal

SAGITTAL VIEW OF ARTERIES OF PELVIS (FEMALE)

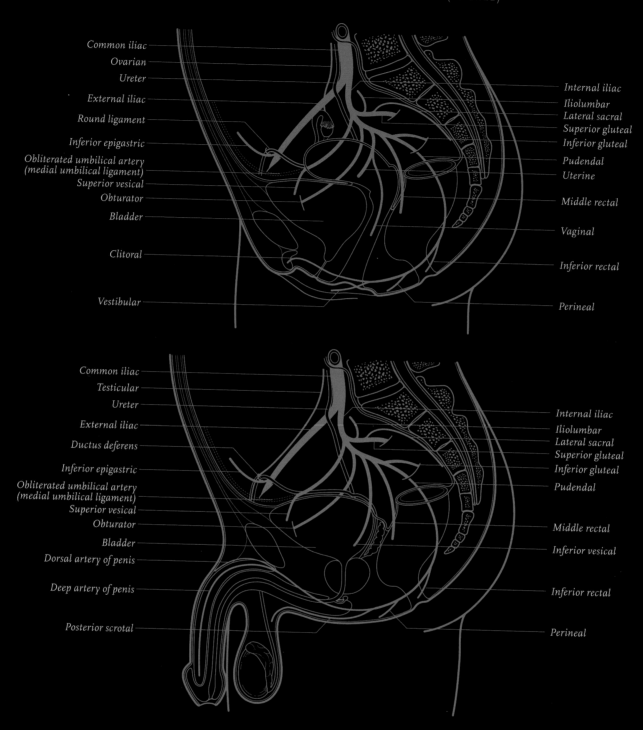

Common iliac

Ovarian

Ureter

External iliac

Round ligament

Inferior epigastric

Obliterated umbilical artery
(medial umbilical ligament)

Superior vesical

Obturator

Bladder

Clitoral

Vestibular

Internal iliac

Iliolumbar

Lateral sacral

Superior gluteal

Inferior gluteal

Pudendal

Uterine

Middle rectal

Vaginal

Inferior rectal

Perineal

Common iliac

Testicular

Ureter

External iliac

Ductus deferens

Inferior epigastric

Obliterated umbilical artery
(medial umbilical ligament)

Superior vesical

Obturator

Bladder

Dorsal artery of penis

Deep artery of penis

Posterior scrotal

Internal iliac

Iliolumbar

Lateral sacral

Superior gluteal

Inferior gluteal

Pudendal

Middle rectal

Inferior vesical

Inferior rectal

Perineal

SAGITTAL VIEW OF ARTERIES OF PELVIS (MALE)

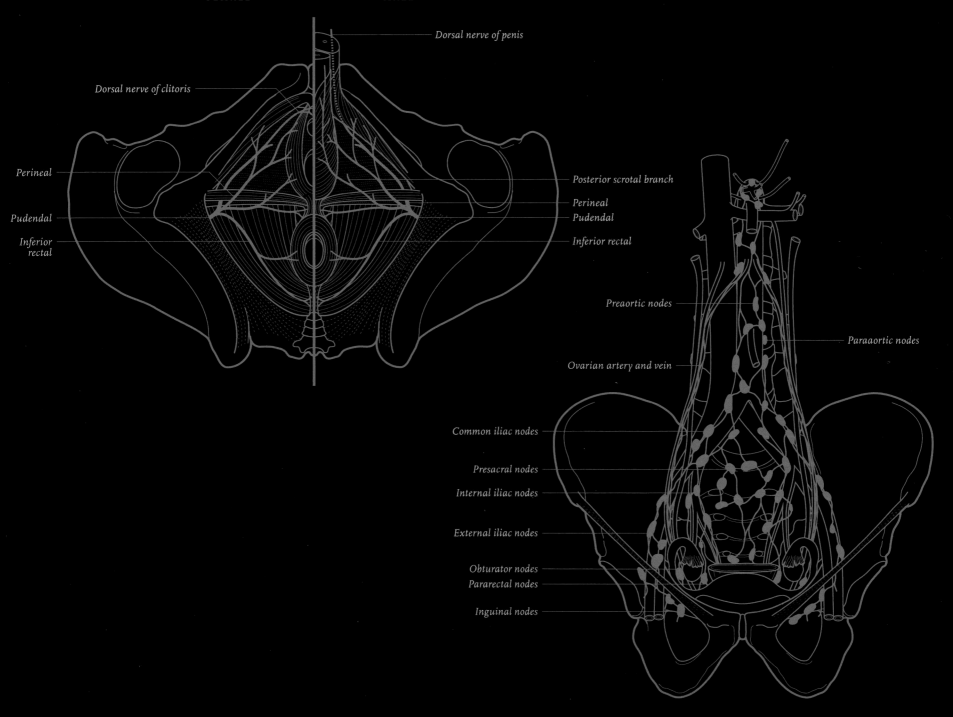

PUDENDAL NERVE IN PERINEUM

FEMALE   MALE

Dorsal nerve of penis

Dorsal nerve of clitoris

Perineal

Pudendal

Inferior
rectal

Posterior scrotal branch

Perineal

Pudendal

Inferior rectal

Preaortic nodes

Paraaortic nodes

Ovarian artery and vein

Common iliac nodes

Presacral nodes

Internal iliac nodes

External iliac nodes

Obturator nodes

Pararectal nodes

Inguinal nodes

LYMPHATICS OF PELVIS (FEMALE)

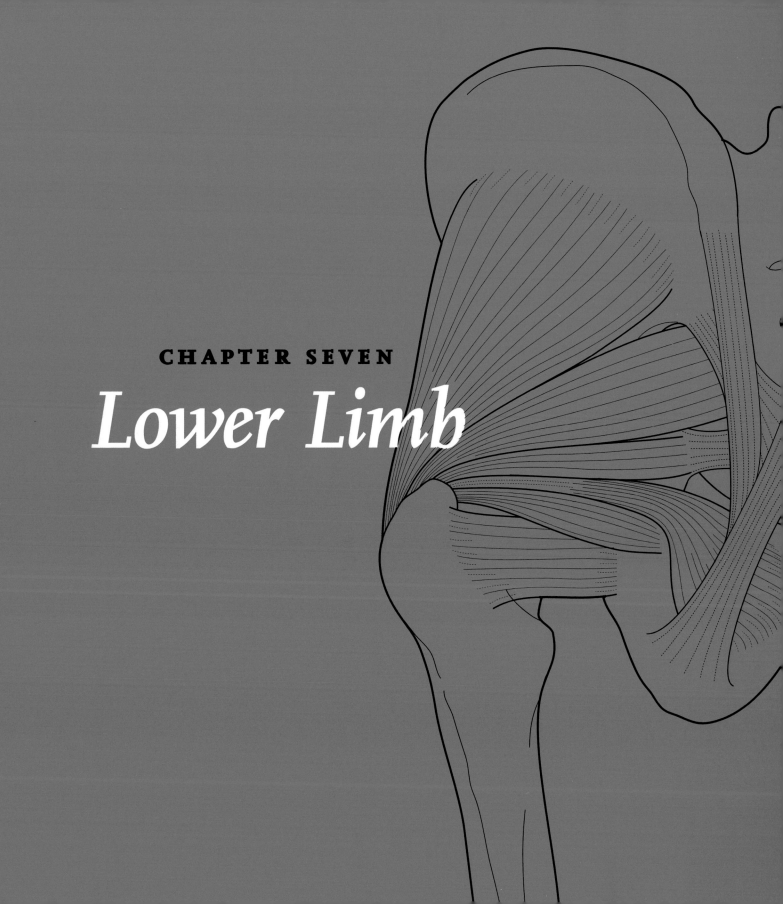

CHAPTER SEVEN
Lower Limb

THE BONES & JOINTS

The lower limb has two main functions: to support the weight of the body and to facilitate locomotion. It can be divided into four regions: gluteal, thigh, leg and foot. The pelvic bone in the gluteal region articulates with the femur of the thigh at the synovial ball-and-socket hip joint between the head of the femur and deep acetabulum of the pelvic bone. The joint is stabilised by this bony congruity alongside capsular ligaments. This stability limits the range of movement to less than that of the upper limb.

The neck of the femur forms an angle of inclination with the shaft, as well as the neck passing backwards from the head to the shaft. These angles support the forwards and upwards thrust involved in locomotion.

The femur articulates distally with the tibia by the medial and lateral femoral condyles on the tibial plateau, and the patella articulates with the anterior surface of the distal femur. This modified hinge joint facilitates flexion and extension of the knee as condyles of the femur glide over the condyles of the tibia, which are deepened by fibrocartilaginous crescent-shaped menisci (meaning 'moon'). Excessive flexion and extension are prevented by cruciate ligaments; the anterior cruciate resists hyperextension, and the posterior cruciate resists hyperflexion. Medial and lateral collateral ligaments further stabilise the knee joint by resisting sideways displacement and excessive rotation.

The second bone of the leg, the fibula, articulates superiorly (by the synovial tibiofibular joint) and inferiorly (by the fibrous tibiofibular joint) with the tibia. Movement is limited as the two bones mostly provide stability for the ankle. Distally, the fibula forms the lateral malleolus and the tibia the medial malleolus.

The seven tarsal bones of the foot are arranged together with the metatarsals to create a weight-bearing arch, reinforced and maintained by plantar ligaments and muscles. The ankle joint is a synovial hinge joint between the distal tibia and the talus bone, permitting plantar flexion and dorsiflexion (extension). The arrangements of ligaments are stronger on the medial side than the lateral side of the joint. Inversion (turning the sole of the foot to face the midline) and eversion (turning the sole of the foot away from the midline) are achieved by the subtalar talocalcaneal and talocalcaneonavicular joints.

The arrangement of metatarsals and phalanges of the foot is similar to the equivalents in the hand, although the first metatarsal is in line with the others and the movements of the phalanges are more restricted.

ANTERIOR VIEW

POSTERIOR VIEW

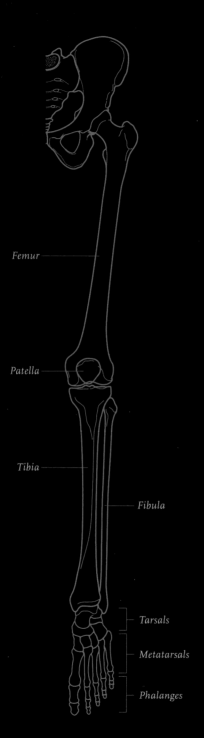

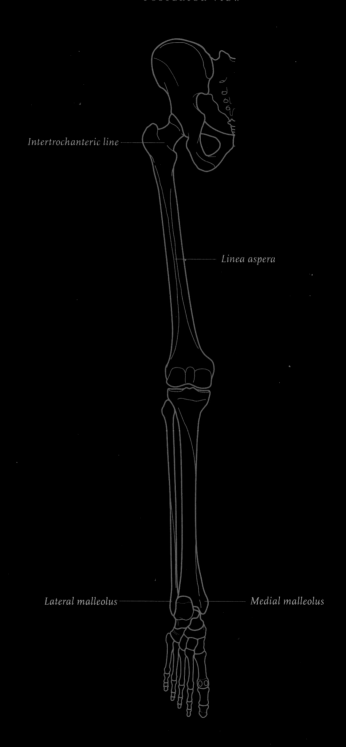

Femur

Patella

Tibia

Fibula

Tarsals

Metatarsals

Phalanges

Intertrochanteric line

Linea aspera

Lateral malleolus

Medial malleolus

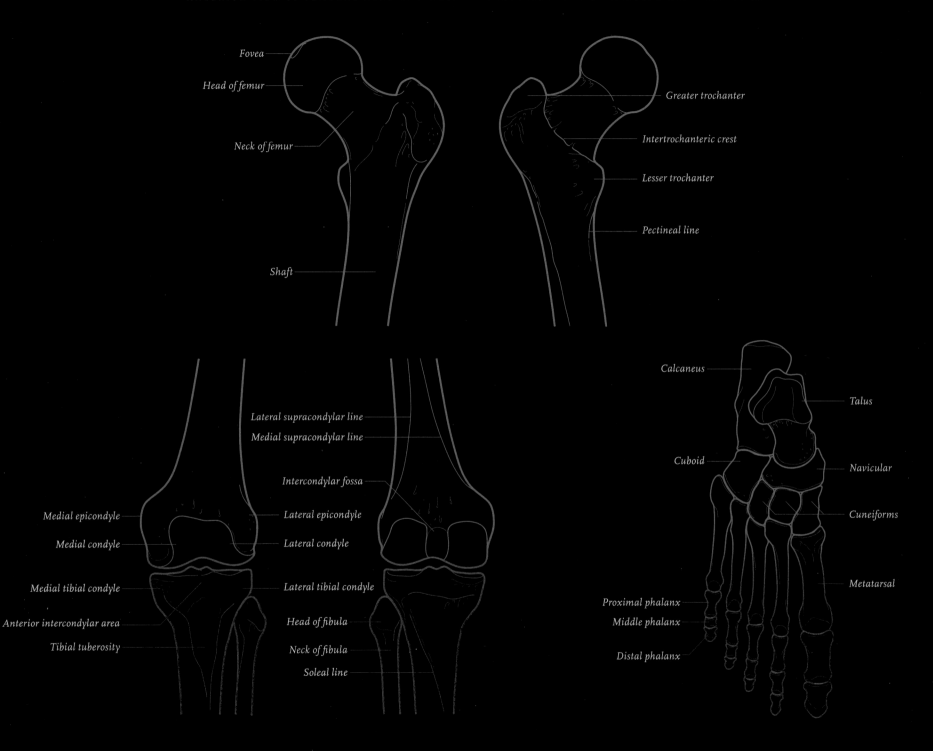

ANTERIOR VIEW OF FEMORAL HEAD AND NECK   POSTERIOR VIEW OF FEMORAL HEAD AND NECK

Fovea

Head of femur

Neck of femur

Greater trochanter

Intertrochanteric crest

Lesser trochanter

Pectineal line

Shaft

Lateral supracondylar line

Medial supracondylar line

Intercondylar fossa

Medial epicondyle

Lateral epicondyle

Medial condyle

Lateral condyle

Medial tibial condyle

Lateral tibial condyle

Anterior intercondylar area

Head of fibula

Tibial tuberosity

Neck of fibula

Soleal line

Calcaneus

Talus

Cuboid

Navicular

Cuneiforms

Metatarsal

Proximal phalanx

Middle phalanx

Distal phalanx

ANTERIOR VIEW OF KNEE   POSTERIOR VIEW OF KNEE   SUPERIOR VIEW OF FOOT

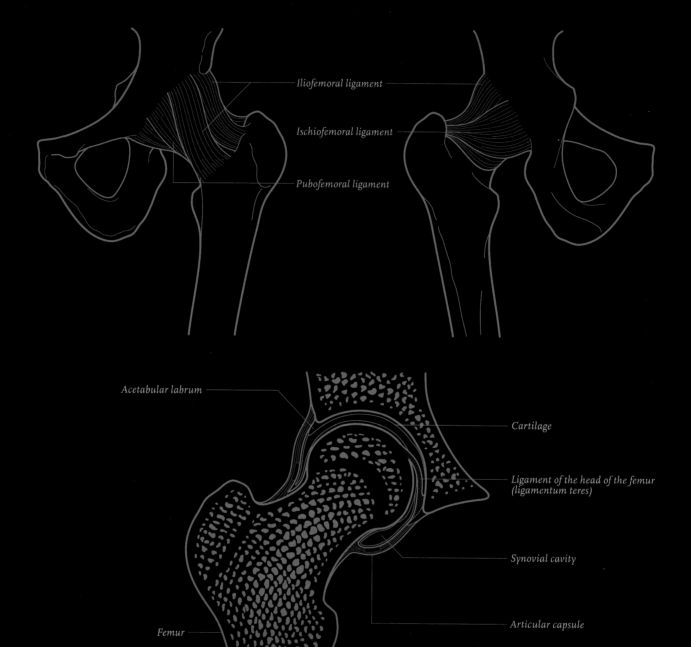

ANTERIOR VIEW OF HIP JOINT

POSTERIOR VIEW OF HIP JOINT

Iliofemoral ligament

Ischiofemoral ligament

Pubofemoral ligament

Acetabular labrum

Cartilage

Ligament of the head of the femur
(ligamentum teres)

Synovial cavity

Articular capsule

Femur

CORONAL SECTION THROUGH HIP JOINT

162

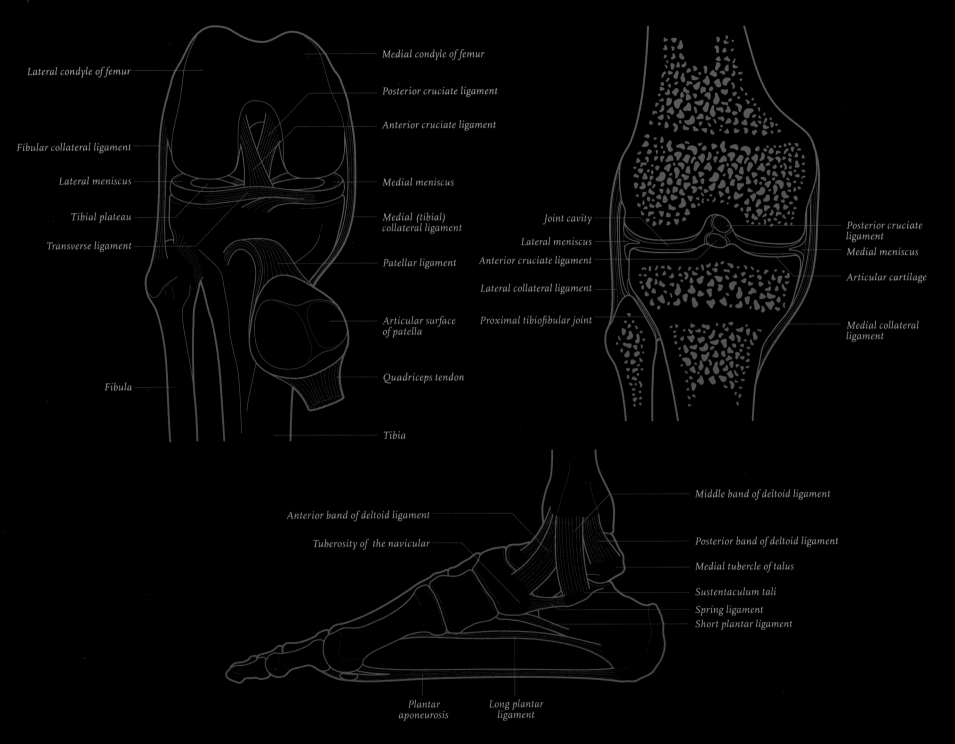

ANTERIOR VIEW OF KNEE JOINT

CORONAL SECTION THROUGH KNEE JOINT

Lateral condyle of femur

Fibular collateral ligament

Lateral meniscus

Tibial plateau

Transverse ligament

Fibula

Medial condyle of femur

Posterior cruciate ligament

Anterior cruciate ligament

Medial meniscus

Medial (tibial) collateral ligament

Patellar ligament

Articular surface of patella

Quadriceps tendon

Tibia

Joint cavity

Lateral meniscus

Anterior cruciate ligament

Lateral collateral ligament

Proximal tibiofibular joint

Posterior cruciate ligament

Medial meniscus

Articular cartilage

Medial collateral ligament

Anterior band of deltoid ligament

Tuberosity of the navicular

Middle band of deltoid ligament

Posterior band of deltoid ligament

Medial tubercle of talus

Sustentaculum tali

Spring ligament

Short plantar ligament

Plantar aponeurosis

Long plantar ligament

MEDIAL VIEW OF FOOT

The bulk of the gluteal region is provided by the three gluteal muscles: gluteus maximus, medius and minimus. All three arise from the ilium, with gluteus maximus also originating from the sacrum, coccyx and sacrotuberous ligament. Gluteus maximus attaches to the gluteal tuberosity on the posterior surface of the femur, and the iliotibial tract together with the tensor fasciae latae muscle. It is a powerful extensor of the hip joint. Gluteus medius and minimus insert into the greater trochanter of the femur. Together they abduct the femur at the hip joint and serve to stabilise the pelvis when the opposite leg is lifted in walking.

Deep to these muscles in the gluteal region is the muscle group collectively known as the lateral rotators. They generally insert into the posterior aspect of the greater trochanter of the femur. Their function is to laterally rotate the extended femur and ultimately the leg and foot during walking.

Laterally, tensor fasciae latae tenses the iliotibial tract into which it inserts, in turn providing stability of the knee joint.

The anterior thigh contains the quadriceps femoris muscle, comprising four muscles: rectus femoris and vastus medialis, lateralis, and intermedius. All four powerful extensors of the knee joint insert into the patella, a sesamoid bone formed within the quadriceps tendon to resist the stress on the tendon. The tendon continues from the patella to insert at the tibial tuberosity as the patellar ligament. Rectus femoris is also a flexor of the hip joint assisting

the iliacus and psoas major muscles, which share a common iliopsoas tendon inserting at the lesser trochanter of the femur. Sartorius also flexes the hip, as well as flexing the knee and laterally rotating the hip. The muscles in the anterior thigh are primarily supplied by the femoral nerve.

Medial to sartorius is the adductor compartment of the thigh. This group of muscles originates from the pelvic bone and inserts predominantly onto the linea aspera on the posterior surface of the femur. Gracilis is an exception to this rule as it inserts on the medial tibia alongside the tendons of sartorius and semitendinosus. It therefore also flexes the knee. Collectively, they adduct the thigh at the hip joint and are innervated by the obturator nerve, except the ischial head of adductor magnus, which is supplied by the sciatic nerve, and pectineus, which is also supplied by the femoral nerve.

The muscles in the posterior thigh are collectively known as the 'hamstrings'. They can extend the thigh at the hip joint as well as flex the knee joint. Originating from the ischial tuberosity (except the short head of biceps femoris), semimembranosus and semitendinosus lie medially and biceps femoris lie laterally. Biceps femoris inserts via a common tendon at the head of the fibula, whilst semimembranosus inserts into the medial tibial condyle, and semitendinosus on the medial tibia with gracilis and sartorius as previously mentioned. The hamstrings are supplied by the tibial nerve, except the short head of biceps femoris, which is supplied by the common fibular nerve.

The posterior leg muscles can be divided into two groups: the superficial muscles (gastrocnemius, soleus and plantaris), which flex the knee and/or plantarflex the ankle, and the deep muscles (popliteus, tibialis posterior, flexor digitorum longus, flexor hallucis longus), which plantarflex the ankle and flex the toes. Tibialis posterior is also an invertor of the foot, together with its anterior component, tibialis anterior.

All of the anterior leg muscles are dorsiflexors (extensors) of the ankle joint, with extensor digitorum longus and extensor hallucis longus also extending the toes.

Muscles in the lateral leg (fibularis longus and fibularis brevis) are principally evertors of the foot, assisted by fibularis tertius in the anterior compartment.

The intrinsic muscles of the foot mostly reside in the plantar region, as those in the dorsum of the foot are two small extensors and four dorsal interossei (abducting the toes). As with the hand, the muscles in the plantar region can be divided into those acting specifically on the big toe (flexor, adductor and abductor hallucis) and the little toe (flexor and abductor digiti minimi). Likewise, there are plantar interossei that adduct the toes, flex the metatarsophalangeal joints and contribute to the extension of the interphalangeal joints. The lumbricals arise from the tendons of flexor digitorum longus and flex the metatarsophalangeal joints while extending the interphalangeal joints.

ANTERIOR VIEW OF GLUTEAL REGION

LATERAL VIEW OF GLUTEAL REGION

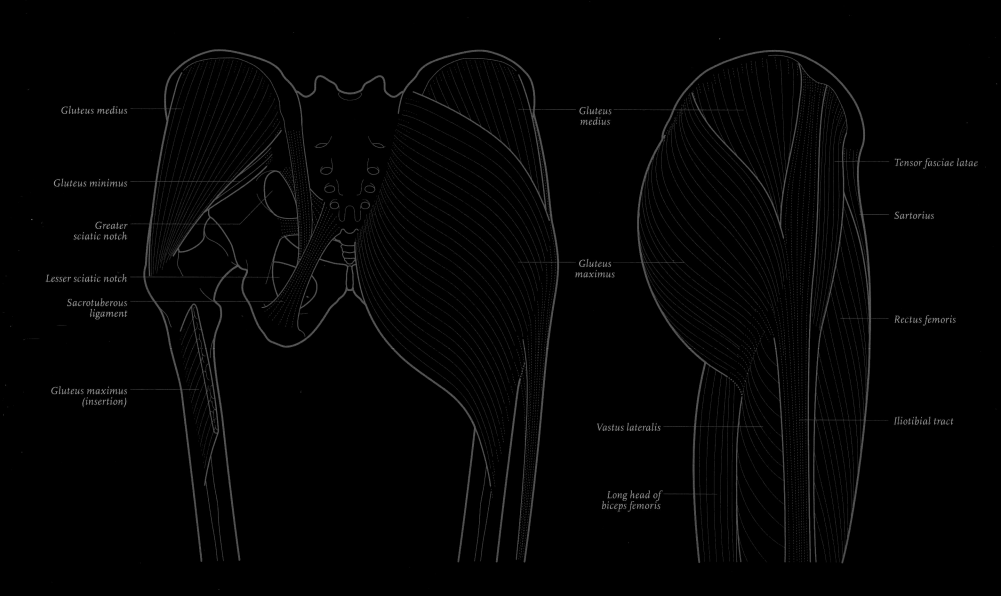

Gluteus medius

Gluteus minimus

Greater sciatic notch

Lesser sciatic notch

Sacrotuberous ligament

Gluteus maximus (insertion)

Gluteus medius

Gluteus maximus

Tensor fasciae latae

Sartorius

Rectus femoris

Vastus lateralis

Iliotibial tract

Long head of biceps femoris

POSTERIOR VIEW OF GLUTEAL REGION

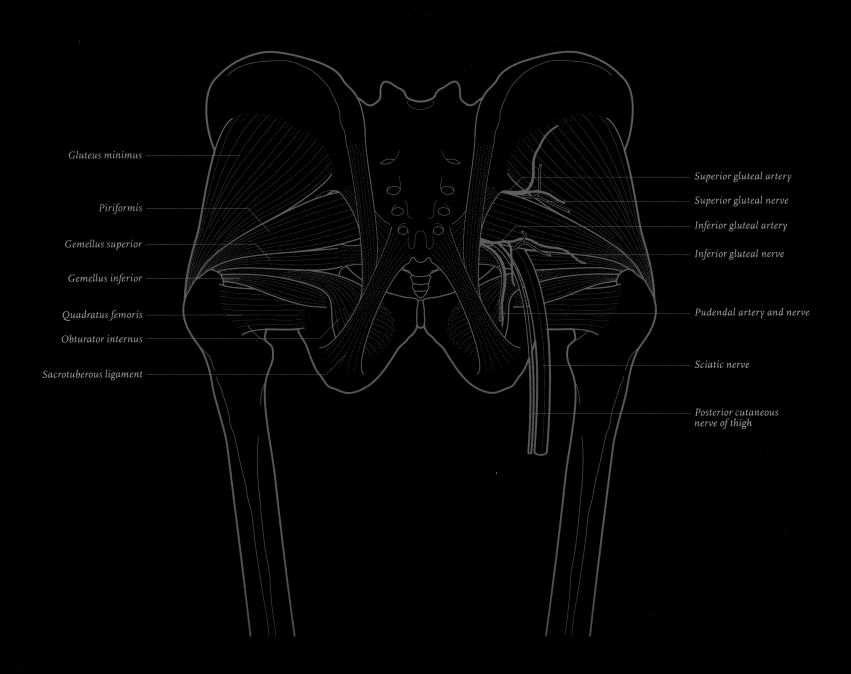

Gluteus minimus

Piriformis

Gemellus superior

Gemellus inferior

Quadratus femoris

Obturator internus

Sacrotuberous ligament

Superior gluteal artery

Superior gluteal nerve

Inferior gluteal artery

Inferior gluteal nerve

Pudendal artery and nerve

Sciatic nerve

Posterior cutaneous
nerve of thigh

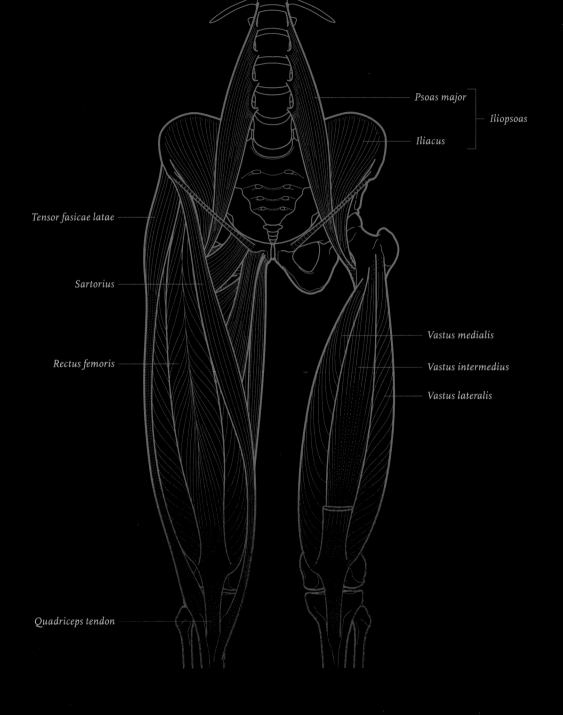

Psoas major

Iliopsoas

Iliacus

Tensor fasicae latae

Sartorius

Vastus medialis

Rectus femoris

Vastus intermedius

Vastus lateralis

Quadriceps tendon

ANTERIOR VIEW OF MEDIAL THIGH MUSCLES

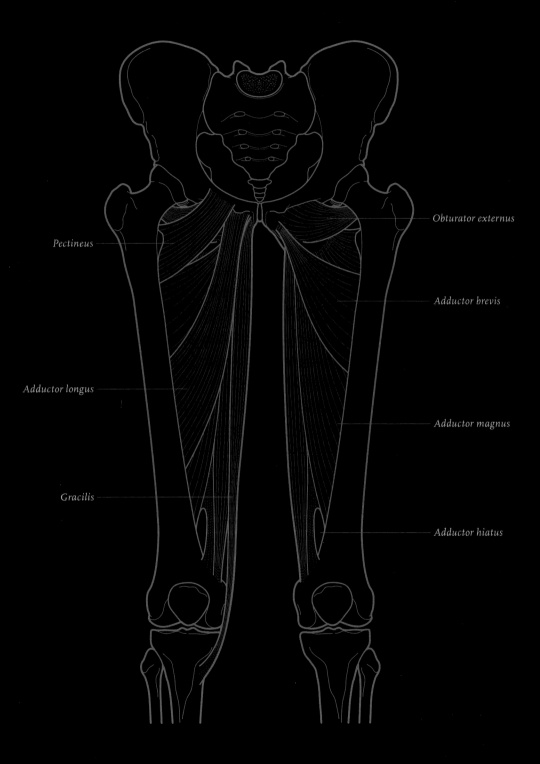

Pectineus

Obturator externus

Adductor brevis

Adductor longus

Adductor magnus

Gracilis

Adductor hiatus

POSTERIOR VIEW OF THIGH MUSCLES

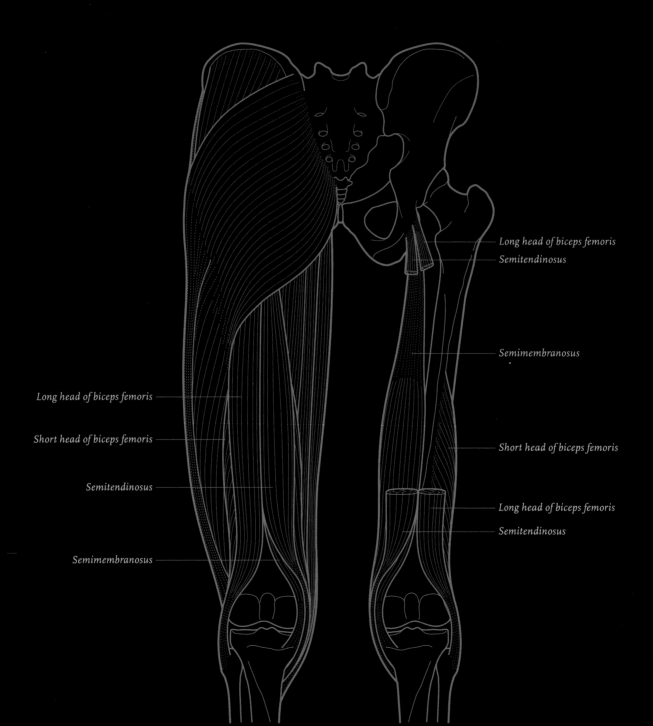

Long head of biceps femoris

Semitendinosus

Semimembranosus

Long head of biceps femoris

Short head of biceps femoris

Semitendinosus

Semimembranosus

Short head of biceps femoris

Long head of biceps femoris

Semitendinosus

TRANSVERSE SECTION THROUGH MID-THIGH

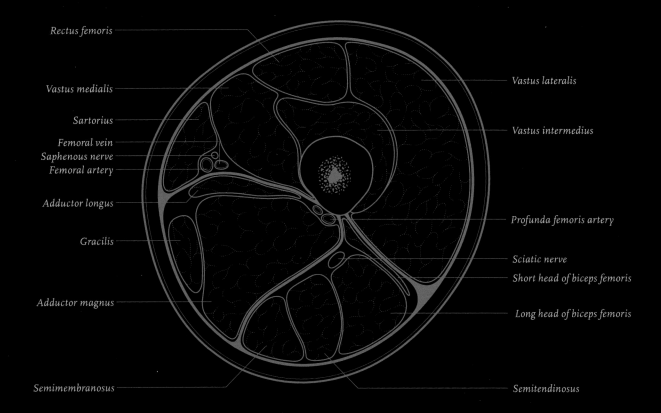

Rectus femoris

Vastus medialis

Sartorius

Femoral vein
Saphenous nerve
Femoral artery

Adductor longus

Gracilis

Adductor magnus

Semimembranosus

Vastus lateralis

Vastus intermedius

Profunda femoris artery

Sciatic nerve

Short head of biceps femoris

Long head of biceps femoris

Semitendinosus

Anterior

Medial ←→ Lateral

Posterior

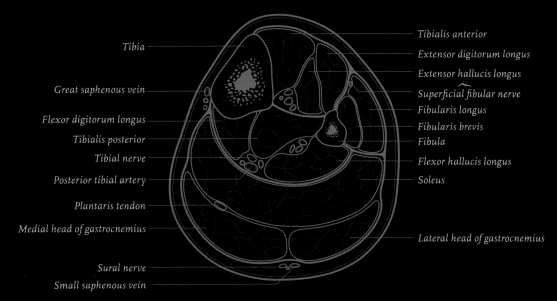

Tibia

Great saphenous vein

Flexor digitorum longus

Tibialis posterior

Tibial nerve

Posterior tibial artery

Plantaris tendon

Medial head of gastrocnemius

Sural nerve

Small saphenous vein

Tibialis anterior

Extensor digitorum longus

Extensor hallucis longus

Superficial fibular nerve

Fibularis longus

Fibularis brevis

Fibula

Flexor hallucis longus

Soleus

Lateral head of gastrocnemius

TRANSVERSE SECTION THROUGH MID-LEG

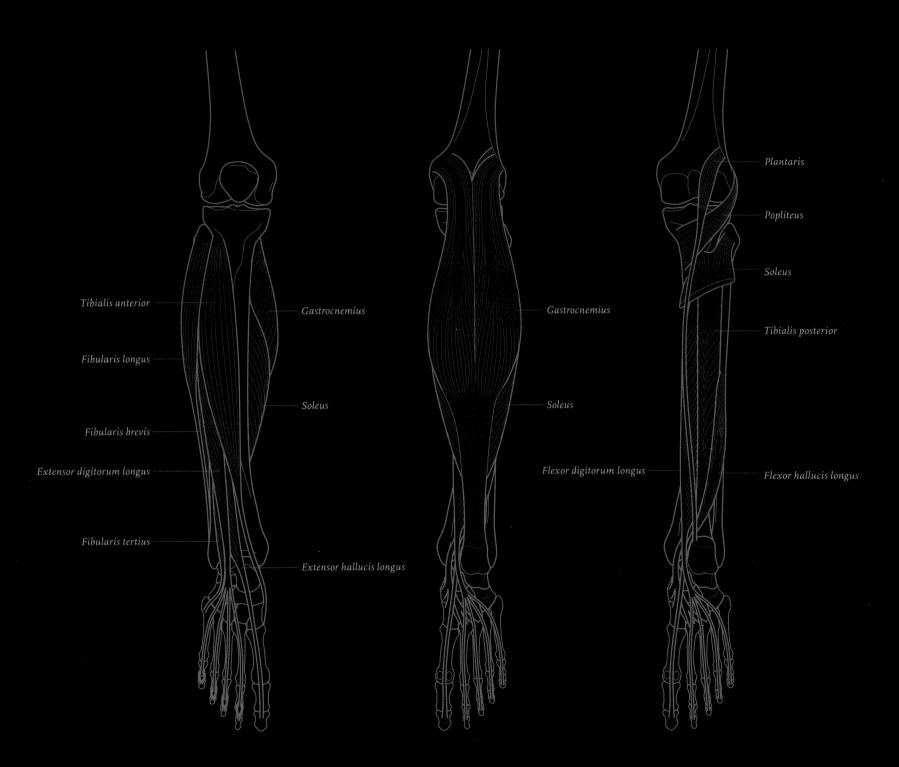

ANTERIOR VIEW OF LEG   POSTERIOR VIEW OF SUPERFICIAL LEG   POSTERIOR VIEW OF DEEP LEG

Plantaris

Popliteus

Tibialis anterior

Soleus

Gastrocnemius

Gastrocnemius

Fibularis longus

Tibialis posterior

Soleus

Soleus

Fibularis brevis

Extensor digitorum longus

Flexor digitorum longus

Flexor hallucis longus

Fibularis tertius

Extensor hallucis longus

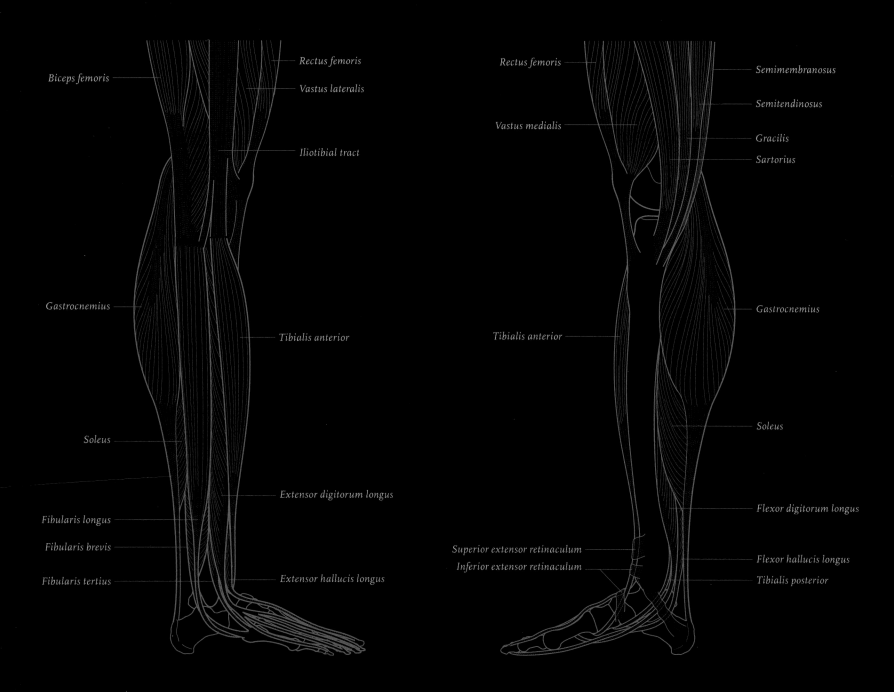

LATERAL VIEW

MEDIAL VIEW

Biceps femoris

Rectus femoris

Vastus lateralis

Iliotibial tract

Gastrocnemius

Tibialis anterior

Soleus

Extensor digitorum longus

Fibularis longus

Fibularis brevis

Fibularis tertius

Extensor hallucis longus

Rectus femoris

Semimembranosus

Semitendinosus

Vastus medialis

Gracilis

Sartorius

Gastrocnemius

Tibialis anterior

Soleus

Flexor digitorum longus

Superior extensor retinaculum

Inferior extensor retinaculum

Flexor hallucis longus

Tibialis posterior

INTRINSIC MUSCLES OF DORSAL FOOT

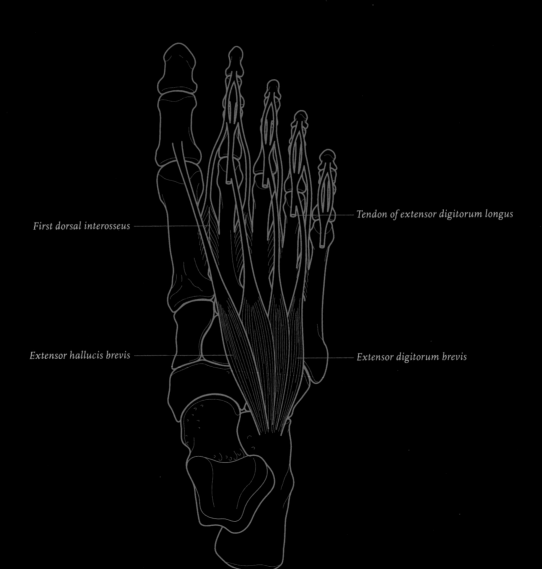

First dorsal interosseus

Tendon of extensor digitorum longus

Extensor hallucis brevis

Extensor digitorum brevis

SUPERFICIAL INTRINSIC MUSCLES OF PALMAR FOOT

DEEP INTRINSIC MUSCLES OF PALMAR FOOT

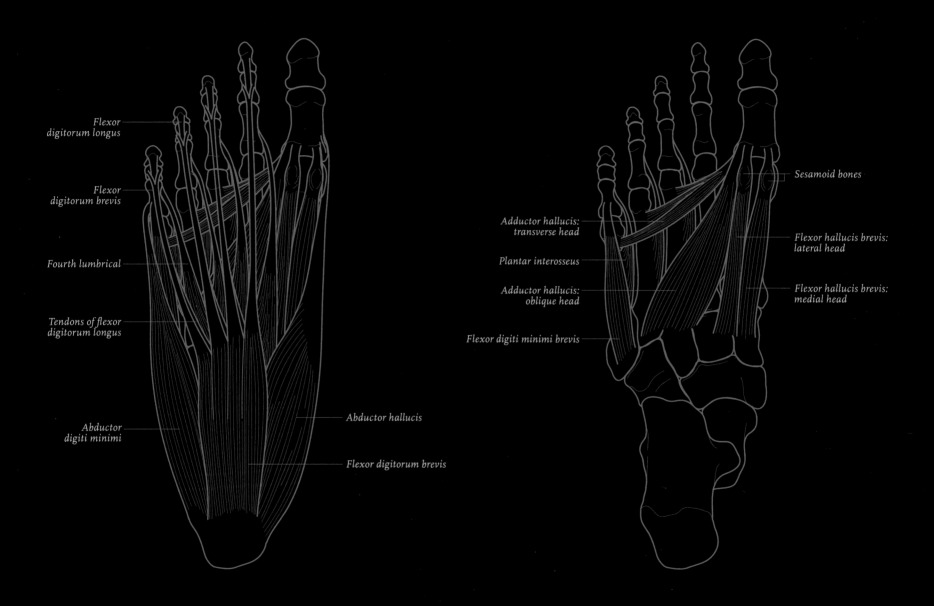

Flexor
digitorum longus

Flexor
digitorum brevis

Fourth lumbrical

Tendons of flexor
digitorum longus

Abductor
digiti minimi

Abductor hallucis

Flexor digitorum brevis

Adductor hallucis:
transverse head

Plantar interosseus

Adductor hallucis:
oblique head

Flexor digiti minimi brevis

Sesamoid bones

Flexor hallucis brevis:
lateral head

Flexor hallucis brevis:
medial head

THE VESSELS & NERVES

The common iliac artery bifurcates into internal and external branches in the region of the sacroiliac joint. The internal branch gives off the superior and inferior branches of the gluteal arteries, which emerge into the gluteal area superiorly and inferiorly to piriformis muscle, as do the corresponding veins, which drain into the internal iliac vein. The external iliac branch continues under the inguinal ligament where it emerges as the femoral artery. This artery of the thigh lies in the femoral triangle alongside the vein medially and the femoral nerve lateral to it in the femoral triangle, surrounded by lymph nodes. After giving off the profunda femoris artery, it continues inferiorly together with the femoral vein, through the adductor canal and pierces adductor magnus muscle at the adductor hiatus, where they emerge on the posterior aspect of the femur as the popliteal artery and vein. Here they can be seen in the popliteal fossa alongside the tibial, common fibular and sural nerves together with popliteal lymph nodes. Genicular branches around the knee ensure that the blood flow is not interrupted with a popliteal

obstruction. Inferiorly, the popliteal artery branches into anterior and posterior tibial branches, which anastomose as the medial plantar and arcuate branches in the foot.

While deep veins flow with the arteries, the superficial veins do not. The dorsal venous arch drains into two veins in the leg. The small saphenous ascends posterior to the lateral malleolus of the fibula, and travels superiorly until it reaches the popliteal fossa, where it joins the popliteal vein. The other, the great saphenous vein, lies anterior to the medial malleolus of the tibia. It continues superiorly throughout the length of the medial leg and thigh, passing behind the knee, until it pierces the deep fascia to drain into the femoral vein in the femoral triangle.

The nerves to the lower limb arise from the lumbar and sacral plexuses on the posterior abdominal and pelvic walls. The spinal nerves of lumbar vertebrae 1–4 form a plexus of nerves behind or within psoas major muscle. The

genitofemoral nerve lies on the surface of psoas muscle and has a femoral branch that is sensory to the skin of the upper anterior thigh. The lateral femoral cutaneous nerve is sensory to the lateral thigh. The femoral nerve supplies the anterior thigh muscles, while the obturator nerve passes along the lateral pelvic wall and through the obturator foramen, to supply the muscles in the medial compartment of the thigh. The sacral plexus gives rise to a number of nerves that supply the perineal and gluteal region, notably the superior and inferior gluteal nerves, pudendal nerve, and posterior cutaneous nerve. The most significant nerve to arise from the sacral plexus is the large sciatic nerve, which emerges from the inferior border of piriformis to travel beneath gluteus maximus into the posterior compartment of the thigh to supply the hamstrings. Just above the knee, it divides into the tibial nerve (supplying the posterior leg and plantar muscles) and common fibular nerve, which supplies the lateral leg by its superficial branch and anterior leg muscles with its deep branch.

ANTERIOR VIEW OF
ARTERIES OF LOWER LIMB

ANTERIOR VIEW OF
VEINS OF LOWER LIMB

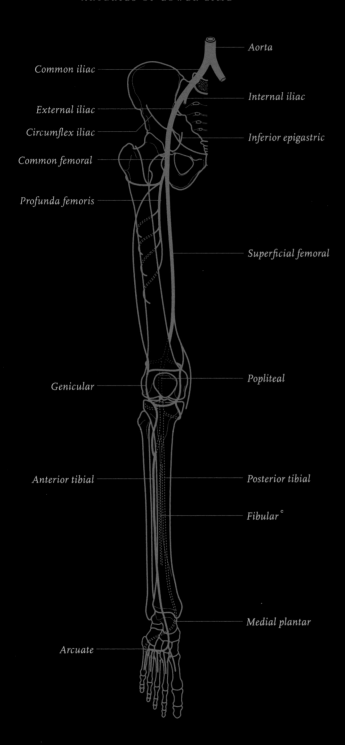

Common iliac

External iliac

Circumflex iliac

Common femoral

Profunda femoris

Genicular

Anterior tibial

Arcuate

Aorta

Internal iliac

Inferior epigastric

Superficial femoral

Popliteal

Posterior tibial

Fibular

Medial plantar

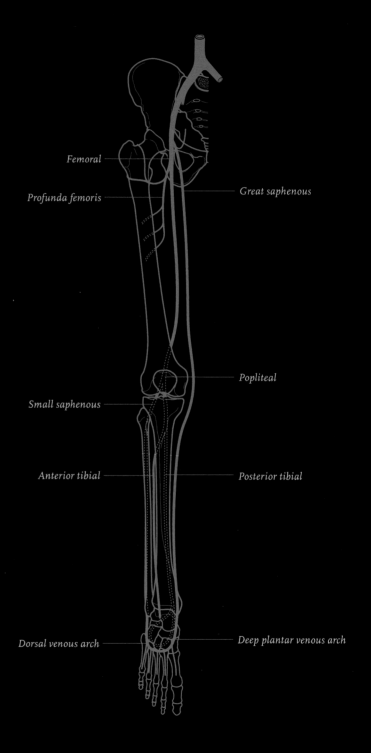

Femoral

Profunda femoris

Small saphenous

Anterior tibial

Dorsal venous arch

Great saphenous

Popliteal

Posterior tibial

Deep plantar venous arch

FEMORAL TRIANGLE

POPLITEAL FOSSA (RIGHT LEG)

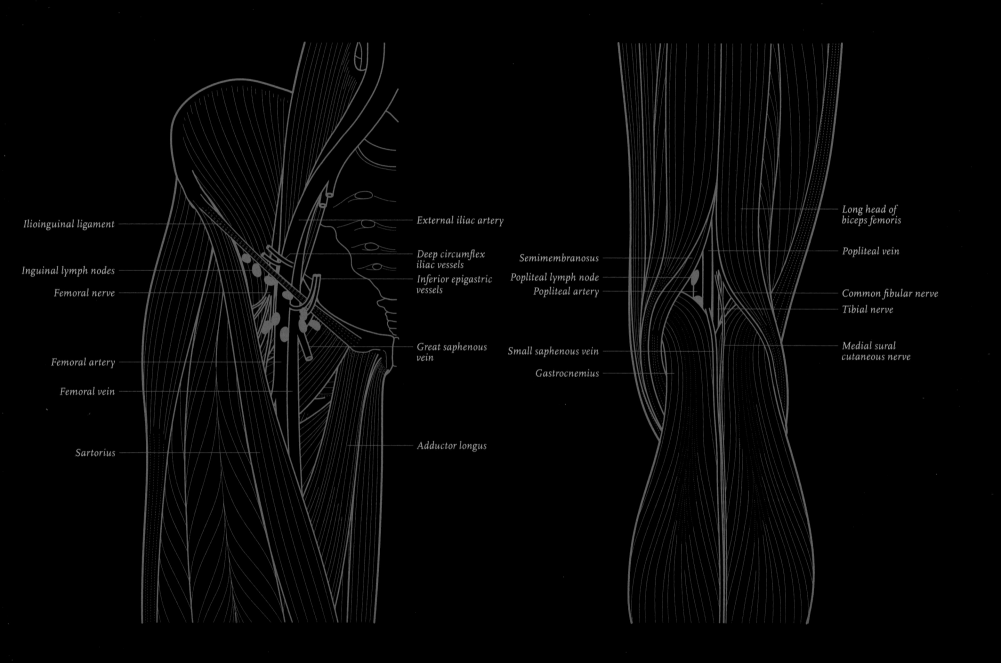

Ilioinguinal ligament

Inguinal lymph nodes

Femoral nerve

Femoral artery

Femoral vein

Sartorius

External iliac artery

Deep circumflex
iliac vessels

Inferior epigastric
vessels

Great saphenous
vein

Adductor longus

Semimembranosus

Popliteal lymph node

Popliteal artery

Small saphenous vein

Gastrocnemius

Long head of
biceps femoris

Popliteal vein

Common fibular nerve

Tibial nerve

Medial sural
cutaneous nerve

179

ANTERIOR VIEW OF LUMBAR & SACRAL PLEXUSES

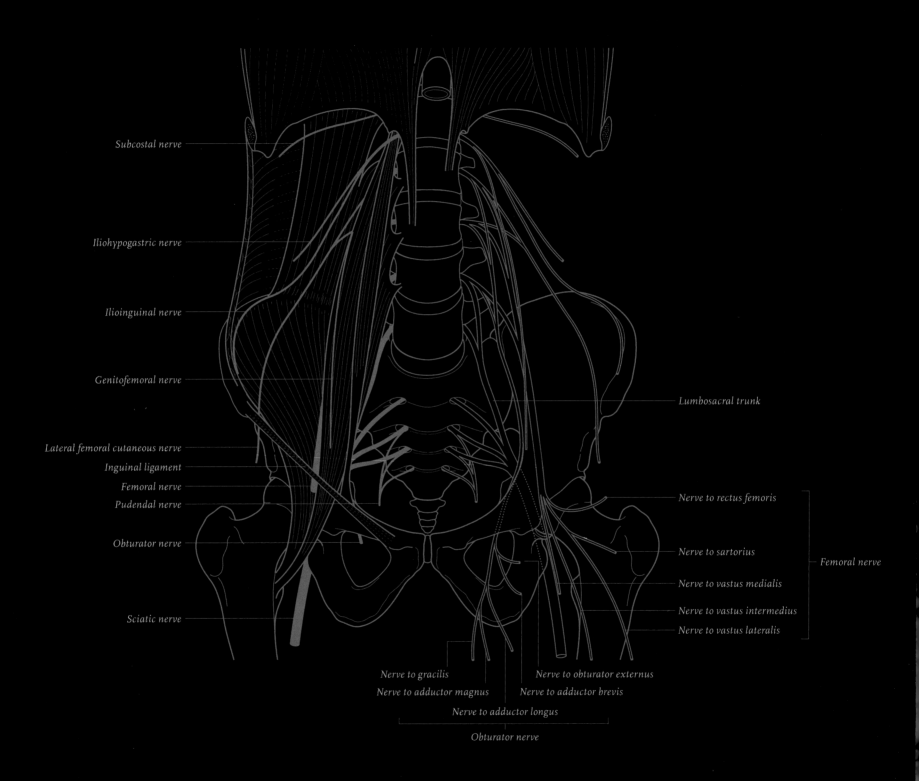

Subcostal nerve

Iliohypogastric nerve

Ilioinguinal nerve

Genitofemoral nerve

Lumbosacral trunk

Lateral femoral cutaneous nerve

Inguinal ligament

Femoral nerve

Pudendal nerve

Nerve to rectus femoris

Obturator nerve

Nerve to sartorius

Femoral nerve

Nerve to vastus medialis

Nerve to vastus intermedius

Sciatic nerve

Nerve to vastus lateralis

Nerve to gracilis

Nerve to obturator externus

Nerve to adductor magnus

Nerve to adductor brevis

Nerve to adductor longus

Obturator nerve

NERVE SUPPLY TO POSTERIOR LOWER LIMB

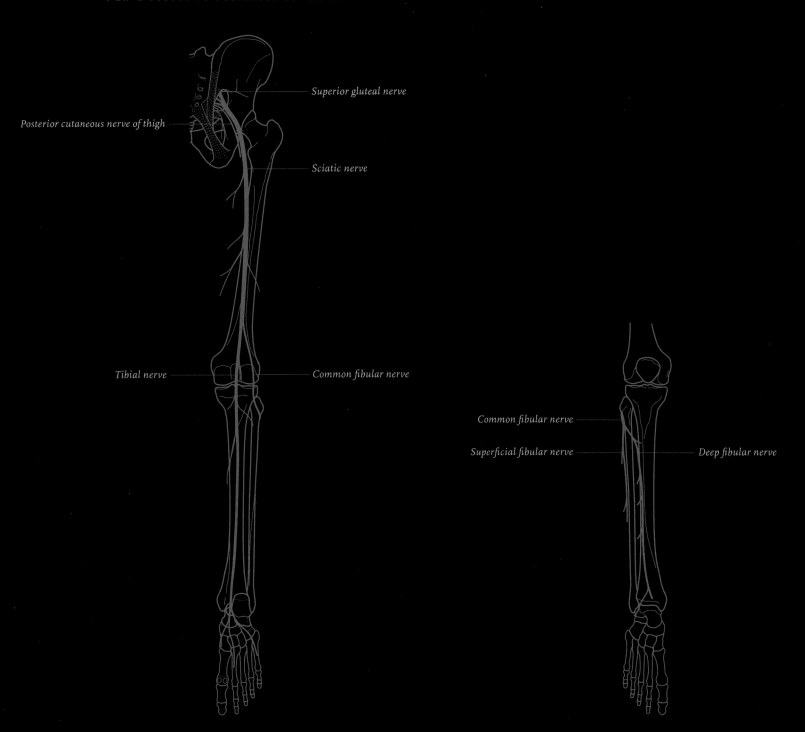

Superior gluteal nerve

Posterior cutaneous nerve of thigh

Sciatic nerve

Tibial nerve

Common fibular nerve

Common fibular nerve

Superficial fibular nerve

Deep fibular nerve

NERVE SUPPLY TO ANTERIOR LOWER LIMB

GLOSSARY *of* ANATOMICAL TERMS

The terminology of anatomy is one that originates from ancient anatomists. Many anatomical words have origins in Greek (Gr.),
Latin (L.) and French (Fr.). The following glossary outlines some of the descriptive words used in this text.

A

Abduct (*L. ab, from + ducere, to lead*)	Movement away from the midline, or fingers and toes from the midline of a body part
Adduct (*L. ad, towards*)	Movement towards the midline, or fingers and toes towards midline of a body part
Afferent (*L. ad, towards + fere, to bring*)	To bring towards. Afferent neurons carry impulses towards the brain
Anastomosis (*Gr. ana, through + stoma, mouth*)	A coming together through a mouth
Anterior (*L. ante, before*)	More in front than another structure in the body
Aponeurosis (*Gr. apo, from + neuron, tendon*)	An expansion of fibrous tissue between a muscle and its attachment
Artery (*Gr. air + terrin, to keep*)	A blood vessel that carries blood away from the heart (thought once to carry air)
Articulation (*L. articulus, joint*)	A joint, a place where bones or cartilages meet
Autonomic (*Gr. autos, self + nomos, law*)	A self-controlled system

C

Carpus (*Gr. karpos, wrist*)	The wrist
Caudal (*L. tail*)	Closer to the feet or lower than any other part
Circumduction	Movement of the distal end of a bone in a circular path while the proximal end remains stable
Condyle (*L. knuckle*)	A rounded knuckle-shaped projection on a bone
Coronal	The longitudinal plane dividing the body into front and back parts
Cortex (*L. bark, shell*)	The outer layer of an organ
Cranial (*Gr. cranion, the skull*)	Of or relating to the skull

D

Deep	Further away from the surface of the body
Depression	Movement that lowers a body part
Distal	Further away from the median plane or root of the limb
Dorsal (*L. dorsalis, back*)	Nearer to the back than another structure in the body, the upper surface of the hand or foot
Duct (*L. ducere, to lead*)	A vessel that brings or leads between parts

E

Efferent (*L. ex, away from + ferre, to bring*)	Away from. Efferent neurons carry impulses away from the brain
Elevation	Movement that raises a body part
Epithelium	Groups of cells that cover or line something
Eversion	Movement of the foot in which the great toe is turned downwards, sole facing laterally
Extension	Straightening motion that increases the angle of a joint

F

Facet (*Fr. little face*)	A small flat surface on a bone
Fascia (*L. band*)	A sheath of fibrous tissue enclosing skeletal muscle

Fissure (*L. fissio, split*)   A groove or cleft
Flexion   Bending motion that decreases the angle of a joint
Foramen (*L. opening*)   An aperture or hole
Fossa (*L. trench*)   A depressed area

G

Ganglion   A group of cell bodies located outside of the central nervous system

H

Hallux (*L.*)   The great toe
Hemi (*Gr.*)   Half
Hiatus (*L.*)   An aperture or opening
Hilum (*L. a spot on a seed*)   An area on a part that marks its point of attachment

I

Inferior (*L. low*)   Closer to the feet or lower than any other part
Inversion   Movement of the foot in which the great toe is turned upwards, sole facing medially

J

Jugular (*L. jugulum, throat*)   The throat or neck

L

Labrum (*L. lip*)   A rim
Lateral   Further away from the median plane
Levator (*L. levare, to lift*)   Movement that lifts
Ligament (*Gr. ligare, to bind or tie*)   Fibrous tissue that joins a bone to its articulating bone
Lymph (*L. lympha, clear water*)   Fluid around cells and tissues carried inside lymphatic vessels

M

Meatus (*L. passage*)   A channel or opening
Medial (*L. medius, middle*)   Closer to the median plane
Median (*L. medius, middle*)   The midline plane dividing the body into right and left halves

P

Papilla (*L. nipple*)   A projection
Parasympathetic (*G. beside*)   Running alongside the sympathetic system
Parietal (*L. parietalis, belonging to a wall*)   Associated with a wall
Phalanx (*Gr. line of soldiers*)   Any of the 14 finger bones or 14 toe bones
Plantar   Of or relating to the sole of the foot
Plexus (*L. braid*)   A network of vessels or nerves
Posterior (*L. post, behind*)   More towards the back than another structure in the body
Pronation (*L. pronus, turned downwards*)   Pivoting movement of the forearm that turns palm downwards
Protraction   Forward pushing movement
Proximal (*L. proximus, nearest*)   Closer to the median plane

R

Retraction   Backwards movement

S

Sagittal (*L. sagitta, arrow*)	The longitudinal plane dividing the body into right and left parts
Septum (*L. sepire, to fence in*)	A partition
Serous (*L.serosus, serum*)	Serum-like fluid
Sesamoid (*Gr. sesame seed*)	A small bone within a tendon
Sigmoid (*Gr. sigma, the letter 'S'*)	'S'-shaped
Sphincter (*Gr. binds tight*)	A circular muscle around an opening to keep it closed
Sulcus (*L. groove*)	A deep furrow on the surface of a structure
Superficial	Closer to the surface of the body
Superior	Closer to the head or higher than any other part
Supination (*L. supinus, turned onto back*)	Pivoting movement of the forearm that turns palm upwards
Suture (*L. suo, to sew*)	A seam
Sympathetic (*Gr. syn, with + pathas, feeling*)	The nervous system that's stimulated in emergency and stress
Synovia (*Gr. syn, with + L. ovum, egg*)	Joint fluid (thought to resemble the white of an egg)

T

Tendon (*L. tendere, to stretch out*)	A strong collagenous fibre that attaches muscle to bone
Transverse	The plane dividing the body into upper and lower segments
Trochanter (*Gr. runner or roller*)	A rounded bony process

V

Vein	A blood vessel that carries blood towards the heart
Visceral	Relating to an internal organ or body cavity

ACKNOWLEDGEMENTS

This book was completed with the invaluable design skills of Alexander James O'Connell, who understood my desire for an anatomy book of beauty and gave precious time to help make my vision become a reality.

I am also indebted to my fellow anatomists and colleagues at Cambridge University, Cecilia Brassett and Michelle Spear, for their expertise and keen eye; Richard Tibbitts and the Medical Artists' Association of Great Britain for their meticulous guidance throughout my medical illustration career; and Vanessa Ruiz and Joanna Ebenstein for joining me in my passion for anatomy and art and supporting my journey.

Finally, many thanks to Jon Hutchings of Lotus Publishing, who has had such faith in my vision throughout the course of this publication, and has allowed me the freedom to create my dream book and aid the publication of this second edition.